LIVING WITH DIABETES

A GUIDE FOR PATIENTS AND PARENTS

LIVING WITH
DIABETES

A GUIDE FOR PATIENTS AND PARENTS

James W. Reed, M.D., M.A.C.P., F.A.C.E.

and

Agiua Heath, M.D.

HILTON PUBLISHING COMPANY   CHICAGO, ILLINOIS

Published by Hilton Publishing Company, Inc.
110 Ridge Road
Munster, IN 46321
815–885–1070
www.hiltonpub.com

Notice: The information in this book is true and complete to the best of the authors'
and publisher's knowledge. This book is intended only as an information reference
and should not replace, countermand, or conflict with the advice given to readers by
their physicians. The authors and publisher disclaim all liability in connection with
the specific personal use of any and all information provided in this book.

Library of Congress Cataloging-in-Publication Data

Reed, James, 1944-
    Living with diabetes : a guide for patients and parents / by James W. Reed and
Agiua Heath.
      p. cm.
    Includes index.
    ISBN 0-9743144-0-4 (pbk.)
    1. Diabetes—Popular works. I. Heath, Agiua. II. Title.
    RC660.4.R435 2004
    616.4'62--dc22   2004021732

DEDICATION

Dr Reed's: To my sister, Idella Whitfield, without whose life-giving gift I would not be alive to write this book. And to my four children, Katherine, Mary, Robert, and David, who remain the brightest stars in my universe.

Dr. Heath's: I want to thank the many colleagues, friends, and family members who read my initial drafts and gave me valuable feedback. I dedicate this book to them and to my patients with diabetes.

CONTENTS

CONTENTS

INTRODUCTION

Eighteen million Americans have diabetes. Due to a combination of hereditary and environmental reasons, African Americans have a higher risk of getting diabetes than the general population. Living with diabetes will require you to make many changes in your life, so finding out you have diabetes can be overwhelming. As with any chronic condition, managing diabetes is a learning process. Once you have learned what there is to know about diabetes, you will be an expert regarding your own body. You can continue to lead an energetic and happy life. Many famous entertainers, athletes, and leaders have achieved great things while managing their diabetes. These include Jackie Robinson, Delta Burke, Elvis Presley, Ernest Hemingway, and B. B. King.

If you or someone you love has diabetes, this book is for you. If you already have been diagnosed with diabetes, this book will help you gain better control. If you are at risk for developing diabetes, this book will help you reduce your risk.

Within these pages, you will learn everything you need to

know about diabetes: from exactly what diabetes is to the reasons why some people are more at risk than others, from the different types of medications available today to the cutting edge advances happening in the field as we write this book, from recognizing and handling emergency situations to understanding the special needs of pregnant women and children, from how to cope with the mix of emotions that comes from having the disease to successful ways to add a healthy diet and regular exercise into your daily routines.

In short, *Living With Diabetes: A Guide for Patients and Parents* will give you the power to take charge of your health—and, ultimately, your life.

Let's begin. . . .

CHAPTER ONE

WHAT IS DIABETES MELLITUS?

Until his wife, Pauline, was diagnosed with diabetes, Stan thought he knew what diabetes was. It was a problem with sugar. But once he learned that Pauline had diabetes, he real-ized he didn't really understand why there was too much sugar in her blood, or how the sugar could hurt her. He went to a diabetes class with her and tried to learn more.

Diabetes Mellitus is also known as "diabetes," "sugar diabetes," or just "sugar."

These words suggest that diabetes relates to sugar. But what is the problem? How do people get it? And what does diabetes do to your body? To understand more about diabetes, you need to understand how your body normally functions.

The *pancreas*, a long, flat organ, lies just behind your stomach. Your pancreas' main job is to help you digest food. When you eat a meal, the pancreas secretes enzymes, which are digestive juices that help break down your food. All food is broken down into protein, fats, or carbohydrates. Carbohydrates are then broken down into *glucose*. (In this book, we will use "glucose" and "sugar" interchangeably for the most part. They are not exactly the same, but they are close enough for what we're going to talk about.)

The pancreas also secretes *insulin*, which helps your body use glucose.

When you eat a meal high in carbohydrates, the pancreas knows to secrete insulin into your blood stream. Once the insulin goes into your blood, it can travel all over your body, telling your body what to do with the glucose. This ability of insulin to affect

Pancreas, Liver, Gall Bladder, and Duodenum with blood circulation system.

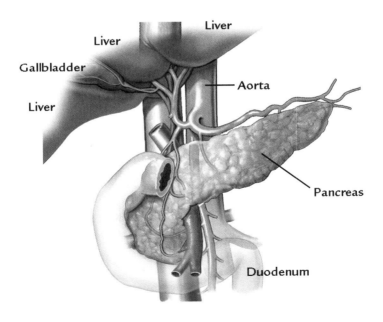

distant parts of your body is what puts insulin in the class of "hormones." *Hormones* are your body's messenger system. Hormones are made in specific organs of the body, such as the ovaries, the pancreas, or the thyroid, for example, and can travel to distant organs to affect changes there. You may have heard of the female hormone, estrogen, and the male hormone, testosterone. Your body makes many others, including insulin.

Think of insulin as a key to unlock cells, allowing glucose to enter. Glucose is our body's main source of energy. Insulin unlocks muscle cells so that they can use glucose for quick energy. Insulin unlocks fat cells so that glucose can enter and be converted to fat. Fat is the body's way of storing and saving energy for later use.

Normally, when our blood glucose increases, so does our insulin. Insulin tells our muscle and fat cells to absorb glucose. Without insulin, these cells will not absorb glucose. Without insulin, liver cells, which can make glucose, will "think" that the body is low on glucose and start the process of making glucose.

WHAT CAUSES DIABETES?

When we have diabetes, the effect of insulin is disrupted. All types of diabetes share the same basic problem: the body doesn't have enough insulin and/or the insulin is not effective. As a result, your body's tissues cannot absorb glucose properly. There is too much glucose in your blood stream, and too little in the body's tissues. This leads to the symptoms and complications of diabetes.

Type 1 Diabetes

There are two main types of diabetes: type 1 and type 2. Less than 10 percent of Americans with diabetes have type 1. We will spend most of this book on the much more common type of diabetes, which is type 2 diabetes. But you should know something about type 1 diabetes as well.

Type 1 tends to happen to children and younger, thinner people. Type 1 diabetes used to be called insulin-dependent diabetes and juvenile-onset diabetes, but these terms are not accurate because people with either type of diabetes might need additional insulin and because both adults and children can get either type of diabetes.

Type 1 diabetes results from the pancreas' failure to produce any insulin. In type 1 diabetes, the insulin-producing cells of the pancreas die, in some cases due to an attack by the immune system. At first, the pancreas produces too little insulin. It eventually stops production completely. Our body depends on insulin to help it use the glucose in our blood stream. Without insulin we can't get our glucose, our body's main source of energy, into our tissues. As a result, our muscles become starved and our blood glucose levels go very high. People with type 1 diabetes must take insulin injections every day or they quickly become very sick and die.

Type 2 Diabetes

The main topic of this book is type 2 diabetes, which used to be called "non-insulin dependent diabetes" and "adult-onset diabetes." These older terms are going out of use, and many children now are getting type 2 diabetes. Type 2 diabetes is the most common type of diabetes, comprising more than 90 percent of cases. It's usually associated with being overweight, but thin people can get it, too. Because more and more people are overweight, type 2 diabetes is increasingly common in both adults and children. People with type 2 diabetes will eventually need insulin.

We saw that in type 1 diabetes the pancreas stops making its own insulin. In type 2 diabetes, the pancreas continues to make insulin, but the body's cells become resistant to the effects of insulin. In our lock and key analogy, this means that although we have the key (insulin) to get in the cells, the lock is jammed. (In type 1 diabetes we have no key.)

In people with type 2 diabetes, the pancreas often produces *more* insulin than normal. However, since their body's tissues are resistant to insulin, the increased amount is still not enough. Later in the course of the disease, the pancreas may make less insulin, but it never stops altogether. Type 2 diabetes doesn't become type 1 diabetes.

Type 2 diabetes can get worse in two ways. First, cells exposed to high blood glucose become more insulin-resistant. So more locks get jammed. Second, with time, our pancreas produces less insulin, and it may eventually stop producing any. We have fewer keys.

Symptoms

The problems in glucose metabolism caused by diabetes affect your entire body. This is why diabetes causes such a wide variety of symptoms and complications. A symptom refers to the way an illness makes you feel. If your glucose is too high, you may get the following symptoms. If you haven't been diagnosed with diabetes, these symptoms should prompt you to be tested. If you have been diagnosed with diabetes, these symptoms suggest that your sugar may be too high.

SYMPTOMS OF HIGH BLOOD GLUCOSE/ SYMPTOMS OF DIABETES

- **Frequent urination**. People developing diabetes often notice that they have to urinate all the time. Blood sugars above the threshold are eliminated by the kidney and causes fluid in the process.

- **Thirst**. People with diabetes also get thirsty because high glucose levels make the blood thick and because of fluid loss in the urine. In response, the brain signals "thirst."

- **Unexplained weight loss**. This is more common in people with type 1 diabetes, but can also happen with type 2 diabetes. It occurs because of loss of sugar (calories) in the urine.

- **Weakness**. Because their tissues are not able to absorb glucose, people lose the energy that glucose provides and feel weak and tired.

- **Blurred vision**. The high blood glucose level causes a shift in the concentration of water in the lens of the eyes, blurring their vision.

- **Hunger**. The lack of glucose-energy makes people feel hungry. This increased hunger can cause people with type 2 diabetes to eat so much that they gain, rather than lose, weight.

- **Yeast infections**. The yeast fungus loves sugar. It thrives when our blood sugars are high. Furthermore, when blood sugar levels are too high, our immune system is unable to work well. Consequently, the body is more vulnerable to yeast infections.

- **Poor healing of wounds**. High blood sugar levels interfere with the body's healing system. As a result, wounds heal slowly or not at all.

WHAT IS DIABETES MELLITUS?

- **Tingling in feet and hands**. High blood sugars can irritate our nerve fibers, leading to abnormal sensations, especially in our feet or hands.

- **Muscle cramps**. These can be a sign of high blood sugar.

- **Cotton-mouth feeling**. This feeling of a dry mouth is a sign of dehydration.

The word "diabetes" is a Greek work for "siphon," referring to the constant flow of urine in people with diabetes. This is how ancient physicians described the sickness that, among other symptoms, made people urinate a lot. These ancient physicians recognized the symptoms of diabetes as well as some of its complications. They even knew that the main problem seemed to be too much sugar in the blood. How? One of them tasted the urine of a person with diabetes and it tasted sweet. This provided the word "mellitus," a Latin word meaning sweet. It was many centuries before physicians understood why some people had so much sugar in their blood. Now we know.

As you can see from its various symptoms, diabetes affects the entire body. However, many people with type 2 diabetes have no symptoms at all. Because of this, millions of Americans with diabetes go undiagnosed. By the time they are diagnosed, 20 percent of people with diabetes have already developed complications. If we can diagnose diabetes earlier, we stand a better chance of preventing complications.

HOW IS DIABETES DIAGNOSED?

In most cases the doctor can do a simple blood test to check for diabetes. He or she may ask you to do a fasting blood test, for which you would prepare by not eating or drinking anything but water for eight hours. This test is usually done first thing in the morning. Your doctor can then check the results within a few hours to a day or so. A fasting blood sugar that is greater than 126 on more than one occasion usually means you have diabetes.

The normal range for blood glucose is less than 100 mg/dl. If yours are in the range of 60 mg/dl to 180 mg/dl, you will need controls.

Laboratory Confirmation of Diabetes:

- Two fasting blood sugar levels greater than, or equal to, 100 mg/dl

- One random blood sugar level greater than, or equal to, 180 mg/dl in someone with symptoms of diabetes

PRE-DIABETES

Before people have type 2 diabetes, they usually have pre-diabetes. Pre-diabetes is defined as a condition in which your fasting glucose is greater than 60 and less than 100. About 20 million people in the United States are estimated to have pre-diabetes.

It's not just numbers. The reason pre-diabetes is important is that even though your glucose is pretty good and you may feel great, the harmful complications of diabetes are already on their way. People with pre-diabetes may already be developing hardening of the arteries and early heart disease. This means that even if you have been told your sugar isn't that high, or you have just "a touch of diabetes," if your fasting glucose is between 100 and 125, you are at risk for complications. People with pre-diabetes can delay or even prevent diabetes by taking steps to improve their blood glucose. We will see how in Chapter 2 when we discuss the Diabetes Prevention Program.

Complications

If diabetes just caused symptoms, you might be uncomfortable, but no more than that. The real problem is that diabetes can cause serious long-term problems, which doctors call "complications."

You have probably heard of many of these. Diabetes greatly increases your risk of having a heart attack or stroke, needing dialysis, losing a foot, or going blind. Many people with diabetes have trouble with pain or loss of sensation in their legs and feet, with their digestion and with sexual function. Because diabetes causes a weakened immune system, people with diabetes are at risk of getting unusual infections and of getting very sick from infections that would not otherwise be dangerous. These complications are serious and frightening, but you can reduce your risk by taking control of your diabetes and of your health in general.

Treatment

Diabetes is a chronic illness. This means that once it has begun, it continues indefinitely. As of now there is no cure for diabetes, but we have more treatments than ever before.

The main goal of treating diabetes is to get your blood glucose as close to normal without having it go too low. Approaching a normal blood glucose level has been proven to greatly reduce your risk of long-term complications. People generally feel much better, too.

There are several treatment approaches to lowering blood glucose. It's always best to change lifestyle first. If you have type 2 diabetes you can improve your blood sugar by reducing your intake of calories, losing weight, and increasing your activity level.

If you have type 2 diabetes you can improve your blood sugar by reducing your intake of calories, losing weight, and increasing your activity level.

You can improve your diet both by eating foods that don't cause your glucose levels to rise as much and by reducing calories to lose weight. Such a diet can lead to better blood sugar levels.

By losing weight, you improve your glucose metabolism. Your cells become more sensitive to insulin, and your blood sugar drops. Exercise is a wonderful way to make your cells more insulin-sensitive. Exercise also helps you lose weight.

As you can see, these lifestyle improvements work together to lower your blood glucose. Continue with them even if you need to take medications. Your doctor can now choose from a wide variety of glucose-reducing medications. We will review them in detail in Chapter Ten.

If the drugs and lifestyle changes cannot sufficiently lower your glucose, your doctor will prescribe insulin. Insulin injections can help reduce your glucose to a safer level. We will discuss the different types of insulin and the ways to administer it in Chapter Ten.

Key Points to Remember

- The pancreas makes insulin.

- Insulin allows our cells to absorb glucose.

- Glucose provides energy for our cells.

- In type 1 diabetes our pancreas doesn't make insulin.

- In type 2 diabetes our cells don't adequately respond to insulin.

- The symptoms of type 1 and type 2 diabetes are similar.

- The complications caused by type 1 and type 2 diabetes are similar and serious.

- We can help prevent diabetes with proper diet and exercise.

- The treatment for diabetes starts with diet and exercise, then progresses to the administration of oral medication and then to insulin.

CHAPTER TWO

WHO GETS DIABETES?

LES WORRIES ABOUT DIABETES

L*es had been on several diets, but always gained the weight right back again. He decided that he was just meant to be big. It kind of depressed him though, because his cousin and his uncle both were overweight and both had diabetes. In fact, his uncle had just suffered a heart attack. Les had read about the rate of diabetes among African Americans and believed that there wasn't much he could do about it. He would probably get diabetes, too.*

But then Les talked to his doctor, who told Les that he could lower his risk of diabetes just by walking every day.

WHO GETS DIABETES?

From 1990 to 2000, the number of American adults with diabetes grew by 50 percent. Most of the increase was due to type 2 diabetes. This increase happened so quickly and was so widespread that diabetes is now being called an epidemic. Why would diabetes suddenly become so prevalent in our society? Researchers believe it's because our unhealthy lifestyle habits are catching up with us.

Most people who develop type 2 diabetes have one or more *risk factors* for the disease. Risk factors are characteristics that indicate that you have increased risk for an illness. None of these risk factors is 100 percent. You could have some of these risks and never get diabetes. You could have none of these risks and get diabetes. But the more risk factors you have the more likely you are to get diabetes.

RISK FACTORS FOR TYPE 2 DIABETES

- Heredity
- Ethnicity
- Obesity
- Body Type
- Inactivity

- Age
- Gestational Diabetes
- Giving birth to a baby weighing over nine pounds
- Polycystic Ovary Syndrome

Type 2 diabetes is hereditary. This means that it can run in families. If your close relative (your parent, sibling, aunt, cousin, or grandparent) has type 2 diabetes, you are more likely to develop it as well.

Type 2 diabetes is more common among certain ethnic groups. Thirteen percent of African Americans, 10 percent of Latinos, and 20 percent of Native Americans have diabetes, compared to 8.4 percent of White Americans. Probably these differences in diabetes rates are mainly due to genetic predisposition, though lifestyle differences play the greatest role.

Obesity is an important risk for type 2 diabetes. Overweight people are more likely to get diabetes. Eighty-five percent of all people with type 2 diabetes are obese. If we can decrease obesity, we will have taken a big step towards decreasing diabetes.

People with an "apple–shaped body" as opposed to a "pear–shaped body" are more likely to get diabetes. "Pear-shaped" people tend to gain weight in their hips. "Apple-shaped" people tend to gain weight in their midsections and have skinny thighs relative to their waists. Being "apple-shaped" may signal that you have *metabolic syndrome* (which we will discuss in Chapter Five). Metabolic syndrome predisposes you to insulin resistance and diabetes, as well as high blood pressure and lipid problems. Both "apples" and "pears" can reduce their risk of developing diabetes by increasing their activity levels and losing weight.

Being inactive predisposes you to diabetes. Physical activity increases insulin sensitivity and keeps your weight at a healthy level. If you are sedentary, that is, if you spend most of your time sitting, you are more likely to develop insulin resistance and become obese, each of which increases your risk of diabetes.

As we age, our chance of developing diabetes increases. Diabetes is more common as we get older. Only 8.7 percent of people age twenty have diabetes, but among people over sixty-five, 20 percent (one in five) have diabetes. The increase in diabetes with age may be due to our pancreas putting out less insulin than before, as well as to us having more fat in our bodies.

Women who have had gestational diabetes have a high risk of developing diabetes.
Women with diabetes during pregnancy, called gestational diabetes, have a high risk of developing outright diabetes later in life. Twenty to 50 percent will develop diabetes within five to ten years.

Women who give birth to a child weighing over nine pounds have a higher risk. Big babies are more common for mothers with diabetes. Having given birth to a big baby can signal a tendency to diabetes.

Polycystic ovary syndrome is an increased risk for diabetes. Polycystic ovary syndrome is an insulin resistance syndrome that can affect women twenty to forty years old. Problems associated with this syndrome include irregular menstrual cycles, weight gain, acne, excess hair growth, and diabetes.

As you can see, some of the risks for diabetes are out of our control; some are in our control. We cannot change our heredity, our ethnicity, or our age. Some people develop diabetes despite being slender, exercising, and eating right. However, experts link the epidemic increase in diabetes to an increase in obesity. Currently, over half of Americans (60 percent) are overweight or obese.

We *can* change our weight, our diet, and our activity levels. African Americans have twice the rate, Hispanic Americans approximately three to four times the rate, and Native Americans up to six times the rate of diabetes than White Americans. Much, but not all, of this increased risk is due to increased rates of obesity among African Americans. Black women have the highest obesity rates in the country. This is due to an interplay of genetics and lifestyle. No one is to blame, but we can do a lot to lower our risk of diabetes by improving our lifestyles. The trick is quite simple: All we must do is improve our diet and increase our activity levels.

We have no time to lose. We are passing down bad habits to our children. Already 18 percent of American children are obese. And rates of diabetes are increasing. One out of three children born in the year 2000 will develop diabetes by age forty if we continue our poor health habits, overeating, and remaining inactive. For black girls the estimate is one out of two! We need to get our children off junk food, super-sized meals, and away from the television set.

African Americans have twice the rate, Hispanic Americans approximately three to four times the rate, and Native Americans up to six times the rate of diabetes than White Americans.

The increase in diabetes is alarming. But knowing the cause shows us the way to a solution. We must reverse the lifestyle problems that lead to diabetes by eating right, getting physically active, and losing any extra weight. This is the way to prevent a genetic predisposition from becoming a disease.

THE IMPORTANCE OF LIFESTYLE

The Pima Indians are one of the Native American peoples in the United States. Their rate of diabetes is one of the highest in the world; half of them have type 2 diabetes!

Interestingly, this is true only among the Pima who live in the United States. Of the Pima who live in Mexico, only 5 percent have diabetes. So in the U.S., 50 out of 100 Pima have diabetes, while in Mexico just 5 out of 100 have diabetes. They are genetically the same people. Why the big difference?

The two groups of Pima have very different lifestyles. When European immigrants settled their land, the American Pima had to move. They stopped living as farmers and fishermen as their ancestors had, and became hunters who ate a diet high in fat and carbohydrates. They stopped being as physically active. In contrast, their Mexican relatives continued their traditional lifestyle, hunting, fishing, eating a diet consisting primarily of beans, vegetables and fruit, and doing daily physical labor. In this case, a change in lifestyle increased the rate of diabetes by a factor of ten!

In Africa, Blacks have a low rate of diabetes because they continue to live a traditional lifestyle of working the land and eating unrefined grains and lots of vegetables and fruit. When they move to the cities, perform less physical work, and eat a more Westernized diet, Blacks gain weight and have increased rates of diabetes.

REDUCING YOUR RISK OF DIABETES

This book will show you how to reduce your risk of diabetes and its complications if you are at risk. If you are at risk for diabetes, we are going to help lower that risk. If you already have diabetes, we are going to help you get it under better control, lower your risk of complications, and get you feeling stronger.

Just as diabetes affects your entire body, dealing with diabetes and getting it under control will require changes in many aspects of your life, but the changes will be for the good. To make those healing changes you will need to learn a lot about diabetes and about yourself.

DIABETES PREVENTION TRIAL

The Diabetes Prevention Trial gives us further encouragement that by changing our lifestyle we can make a difference. In it, people were able to improve their lifestyles and prevent diabetes. In the Diabetes Prevention Trial researchers studied Americans of various ethnicities who were at high risk of developing diabetes. They compared people who continued their previous lifestyles to people who improved their diet, increased their activity levels, and lost a moderate amount of weight. This second group exercised for a half-hour each day, five days a week, and lost an average of ten pounds. After two years the researchers found that the group who walked regularly and had lost weight was 60 percent less likely to develop diabetes.

How did this group improve their health so much? They increased their physical activity with the mild exercise of walking for only two-and-a-half hours each week. They also ate better diets. The researchers called this "lifestyle balance." We all need to pay attention to both exercise and diet. The people who reduced their risk of diabetes were just regular people from all ethnic and racial groups who needed help and support, which they received through the research program.

Changing your lifestyle is not easy. You will need a strategy, and you will probably need support from others, but it is certainly possible. And the rewards are worth it: you will feel better and more than likely live a longer, healthier life.

LES TAKES IT ONE STEP AT A TIME

Les decided to get more information about lowering his risk of diabetes. He took a class at his local hospital. He learned how to increase his activity level and how to eat better. Although starting a new diet made him think of the failures he'd had with old diets, Les stuck with it.

As to his activity level, Les took it slowly. He began walking every day for half an hour, and getting off the bus one stop early on his way to work. He also put away the remote for the TV. That way, he was forced to get up and stretch if he wanted to change the channel. Finally, he stopped eating out and didn't buy any snack food.

Prevention

The Diabetes Prevention Program showed us that lifestyle changes could prevent high-risk people from actually developing diabetes. If you have one or more of the risk factors we discussed, you are at high risk. In this case, you should get *screened* for diabetes. Being screened means getting a test to see if you have a disease even though you have no symptoms of the disease. This means getting a fasting glucose test, as we discussed in Chapter One. Twenty percent of people diagnosed with diabetes already have complications at the time of diagnosis. If we can diagnose diabetes and pre-diabetes earlier, we stand a better chance of preventing complications.

A Healthier Family/A Healthier Community

As adults, our behavior powerfully influences our children and our families. Once you improve your diet, you will be helping your children improve theirs. But we hope that the healthy lifestyle will spread throughout our society. Given the powerful results of the Diabetes Prevention Trial and the alarming increase in diabetes among Americans, we should work on improving the health habits of our communities as a whole.

What to Remember About Your Risk of Developing Diabetes

- Some risk factors are fixed: heredity, ethnicity, and age.

- Some risk factors can be improved: weight, diet, and activity level.

- Improving your lifestyle by eating right, exercising for half-an-hour, five days a week, and losing weight can lower your risk for developing diabetes.

- If you have risk factors for diabetes, you should get a screening test.

CHAPTER THREE

DIABETES IN YOUR CHILD

MARY'S SON GETS DIABETES

Mary was worried about her twelve-year-old son, Daniel. He had just gotten over a virus and now he seemed to have stomach flu. He kept vomiting and crying that his tummy hurt. Mary became so concerned that she took him into the ER to make sure it wasn't his appendix. She was stunned to hear that Daniel had diabetes and would have to be on insulin for the rest of his life. She didn't believe the doctor. She was a single mom. How would she ever be able to deal with a diabetic son!

Diabetes is the most common chronic disease of childhood next to asthma. In the United States alone, 130,000 children have diabetes. Many more have diabetes and don't know it. In the past, over 90 percent of adult diabetics had type 2 diabetes; children almost always had type 1 diabetes. (In fact, type 1 diabetes used to be called "juvenile-onset diabetes" and type 2 diabetes used to be called "adult-onset diabetes.") However, since 1970, the rates of childhood obesity have tripled and more and more children are developing type 2 diabetes. Now, 40 percent of diabetic children have type 2 diabetes.

TYPE 1 DIABETES

Type 1 diabetes occurs when the pancreas no longer makes insulin (*See Chapter One*.) The insulin-producing cells of the pancreas die, in some cases, due to an attack by the immune system, usually after a viral illness. As the insulin-producing cells die, the pancreas produces less insulin. Eventually insulin production stops completely. Without insulin our cells can't absorb glucose—their main source of energy. With glucose trapped outside cells, they are deprived of energy, and blood glucose rises to dangerous levels.

Although type 1 diabetes can affect children as young as newborns, the typical onset is around puberty. The average age for girls is 10–12, for boys, 12–14. (Type 1 diabetes can have its onset in older persons too. For example, alcoholics who suffer from bouts of pancreatitis can get type 1 diabetes, as well as adults with pancreatic cancer or with certain infections that can affect the insulin-producing cells of the pancreas.) Type 1 diabetes is less common in African Americans than in White Americans.

The symptoms of type 1 diabetes are similar to those of type 2 diabetes, but because type 1 is due to the absence of insulin, its onset tends to be more dramatic. Weight loss, vomiting, and stomach pain are more common in type 1 diabetes.

Other possible symptoms are:

• Frequent urination

• Thirst

- Sugar cravings

- General hunger

In a baby or toddler, the symptoms of diabetes can be difficult to detect. Frequent urination is easy to miss in a child who isn't toilet-trained and who can't tell you what's bothering him. Often a baby becomes quite sick before parents realize that he's not just having a virus.

IS IT TYPE 1 OR TYPE 2?

When diabetes starts, it's sometimes difficult to know which type it is. The doctors might suspect either type 1 or type 2, but they may not be sure; although people with type 1 diabetes eventually have no insulin, they may still have a little as their insulin-producing cells die off. Also, as people develop diabetes, their pancreas may work extra hard to put out insulin, causing a brief improvement in their blood glucose control. This time when blood glucose improves is called the *honeymoon period*. This period makes people hope that their diabetes is going away, but that never happens.

Anyone developing diabetes should be in especially close contact with his health care provider. Initial medication requirements can change quickly.

TYPE 2 DIABETES

Type 2 diabetes occurs when our cells become resistant to insulin. In children, this is always associated with obesity. Fifteen percent of children in the United States are now seriously overweight. This rate has tripled since 1970. Like adults, children have been getting less exercise and eating too much. Many children spend most of their free time sitting in front of a TV set. Schools have cut back on recess time and on athletic programs, leaving children with fewer opportunities for physical activity. Combine the rise in obesity with a genetic predisposition, and, chances are, diabetes rates will increase.

But genetic risk factors are also responsible. Roughly 60 percent of children with type 2 diabetes have a parent with diabetes. Most are from ethnic minorities. Two-thirds are girls.

Diabetes is more serious for children. They have their entire lives ahead of them, giving them more years with diabetes to develop complications.

Symptoms of Type 2 Diabetes

Type 2 diabetes generally starts more subtly than type 1. A significant number of children with type 2 diabetes don't even know they have it. Symptoms to look for include:

- Frequent urination

- Thirst

- Blurred vision

- Infections

- Weight loss

A DIABETES-RELATED CONDITION

Acanthosis nigricans is a condition characterized by dark skin tags in the armpits and on the neck. It is seen in 60 percent of children with type 2 diabetes.

CHESTER WORRIES ABOUT HIS DAUGHTER

Chester had been worried about his 13-year-old daughter, Tamika, for a while. Ever since they'd moved to a new town, she seemed depressed. She wasn't doing too well in school, and, on weekends, she just sat in front of the TV and ate potato chips. Chester thought Tamika was beautiful, but she was getting kind of chubby. When she started complaining about blurred vision and refusing to go to school, Chester believed she just wanted to avoid her classmates and their teasing. But he took her to the doctor just to be sure. He was stunned when the doctor said it was diabetes. Chester had had diabetes for years; he should have seen the signs!

DEALING WITH DIABETES IN YOUR CHILD

Finding out your child has diabetes is a shock. But, as a parent, you need to get a grip on your feelings so that you can best help your child. You will need to provide your child with a healthier lifestyle, including a better diet and increased physical activity. You may be called upon to do glucose checks, or, if your child is older, check that the child does them herself. You may need to administer insulin injections or monitor your child as she takes her medication. For a busy parent, all these new responsibilities can seem overwhelming.

Your child may be going through the emotional turmoil that occurs when you find out you have diabetes (*See Chapter Four.*) However, since she is a child, she probably has less wisdom to draw upon to make sense of things. You will have to comfort her—while also dealing with your own feelings of sorrow and guilt. Many parents feel guilty when their child is diagnosed with a chronic illness. They worry that it is their fault. It is *not* your fault. The reasons that people get diabetes are complex. It is never just heredity or just diet or just becoming overweight. So don't blame yourself that your child has diabetes. On the other hand, do take responsibility now for helping your child live as healthily as possible.

Another source of guilt and stress for a parent is weighing the needs of the child who has diabetes with the needs of the rest of the family. It is normal to have to devote more attention to the child with diabetes, especially just after the diagnosis. The two of you need to learn all about the disease and how to treat it. You will need to take tests and go to doctors' appointments. You will have to figure out how to make the lifestyle changes that will be necessary for your child to avoid complications. It makes sense that other family members might feel left out or neglected.

MAKE YOURS A HEALTHIER HOUSEHOLD— IN EVERY WAY

Food

Nobody in the family will appreciate having to eat a more restricted diet. This can leave you feeling conflicted. But, if you continue to have snacks and sweets in the house, it makes the child with diabetes feel left out. On the other hand, if you get rid of the snacks and sweets, your other children will be unhappy. Please remember that a healthier diet is best for *everyone* in the family. It will help support your child with diabetes and it will help your other children lead healthier lives. Remember, diabetes is inherited. You want to do all you can to prevent diabetes in your other children. A healthy diet not only reduces their risk of diabetes, but also obesity, heart disease, high blood pressure, high cholesterol, cavities, and cancers. It is likely to help them grow stronger and to have more energy. Your job, as the parent, is to do what is best for them, not necessarily what they like.

Physical Activity

The entire family should increase their physical activity level. Limit TV viewing time. Children who spend hours in front of the television set or computer terminal don't get as much exercise as they need. Increase your awareness of how television advertising influences you and your children. Advertising is a multi-million dollar business whose aim is to convince people that they want a product. The ads make what they are selling look very desirable; your children may feel they won't be happy or popular if they can't have that product. Unfortunately, much of the food advertising directed at children is for unhealthy foods. Overly-sweet cereal, drinks, snacks high in fat and salt, and fast food are all made to seem very cool. You either need to turn off the TV or make sure your children understand that they don't need to consume what's advertised on the tube to be healthy and happy. Please note: while encouraging your diabetic child to get physical activity, also make sure to check their sugars before and after activity. This is important because your child should not exercise if her sugars are low.

Younger Children

If your diabetic child is small, your job will be easier because you have more control. You can choose a healthy diet for him or her. Almost everybody likes fat, salt, and sugar, but you can train your taste buds to enjoy less of these. For example, whole milk seems too greasy and heavy to people used to low fat milk. If you start your child off on a healthy diet, your child is more likely to enjoy healthier foods in the future.

It's hard for children to be as organized as the demands of diabetes requires. Help them stay on a schedule of healthy meals and snacks, regular exercise, and medication as needed.

Once they are in the habit, children as young as seven can learn to check their sugars and administer their own insulin. This can help them feel independent and in control. At a younger age, children are less susceptible to peer pressure. Their friends might even think that their glucose meter is "cool." Give your child the message that he is a normal, powerful person. He can do everything a child without diabetes can do, with minor modifications to care for his health.

Hypoglycemia

If your child is on medication, the entire family should know how to recognize and treat hypoglycemia.

The early symptoms of hypoglycemia are the same in children as in adults. (*See Chapter Seven.*) They are:

- Feeling shaky

- Breaking into a cold sweat

- A rapid heartbeat

- Feeling faint

- Feeling clumsy

- Sudden hunger

- Sudden fatigue

- Headache

If your child is too young to communicate to you, look out for changes in mood and level of alertness.

Keep glucagon (prescription-only vials of the hormone that causes the liver to release stored sugar) at home and make sure the entire family knows how to use it, and that they know when it's time to call 911. (*See Chapter Seven.*)

Until your child reaches adolescence, it's better to let his sugars be a little high than on the low side. For young children, hypoglycemia is less of a concern. Studies have shown that the most important time to control sugars to avoid diabetic complications is when children enter their teens. At that point, it's time to move to tighter control.

In School

If your child is old enough to go to school, you are entitled to get help from the system. Diabetes is considered a disability; it is illegal to discriminate against someone with diabetes. This means that, in school, your child is entitled to participate in all school activities. In addition, the school must give your child the opportunity to care for her diabetes. The school must allow her to have necessary snacks, go to the bathroom, test her blood glucose, and take her medication. She is entitled to get help with these functions if she needs it. School staff that are in contact with your child need to be able to recognize and treat hypoglycemia.

Educate yourself as to what foods are available at the school. Many school lunches and school vending machines provide too much food that's high in fat, sugar, and salt. If this is the case, your child will need to bring her own food. (You are responsible for any supplies she needs.) Better yet, work with the school staff and other parents to improve food selection for all children. You can get advice on how to do this from the School Foods Tool Kit manual put out by the Center for Science in the Public Interest (CSPI), a nutrition advocacy group. The School Foods Tool Kit is available online at *http://cspinet.org/schoolfood*.

Look into a diabetes camp. They are located throughout the country and specialized in activities for diabetic children. At diabetes camp, your child will learn to take care of his diabetes. He will live a healthy lifestyle, check his sugars, eat right, and exercise. Maybe even more importantly, he will meet other children just like him, and feel less alone. This is a wonderful experience for kids with diabetes.

Your Teenager

The teenage years bring new challenges to the treatment of diabetes in your child. During this time, it's normal for children to want to fit in with their friends and to separate themselves from their parents. As a result, your child may want to deny the fact that she has diabetes (unless her friends have it, too). She may stop taking her medication and eating properly. Some girls go as far as developing eating disorders and try to skip their medication to lose weight.

Being a teenager is a time of strong emotions and many teens are prone to depression. Overweight children tend to be made fun of by their peers. If your teen is overweight, she may feel isolated—and stay isolated because she feels different. This can lead to your teenager avoiding activities and staying home to watch TV and eat.

Try to keep the lines of communication open. Spend time together. Prepare meals together. Go for walks.

Make sure your teen knows about safe sex and birth control. A baby born to a teen mom who didn't control her diabetes ahead of time will not have a good start in life. Live a healthy lifestyle yourself, so that your teen has you as a good example.

Healthy Lifestyle Choices for Kids and Teens

- Water and nonfat milk are healthiest, and diet sodas are a good alternative to soda pop.

- Don't "super-size" it.

- Have your child learn which foods are healthier.

- Give your child healthy snack alternatives.

- Feed your child's self-esteem.

- Encourage physical activity.

- Limit TV viewing.

CHAPTER FOUR

DEALING WITH YOUR FEELINGS

ANGELA GETS THE NEWS

When Angela, a young, vivacious sales woman, was diagnosed with diabetes, she was really annoyed. She had just been promoted at work. She was dating and trying to find someone to marry. She was working so hard to be a success, and now diabetes had come around to ruin her life! She was disappointed in her doctor. He used to be warm and respectful. Now, suddenly he had become too serious, trying to scare her by talking about blindness and kidney failure. His nurse had assured her that her sugar wasn't really that bad. Angela simply didn't trust the doctor.

At the office Christmas party, she avoided the desserts by telling people that she was on a new diet. She wasn't going to let anyone know she had diabetes. In fact, she wasn't sure she even had diabetes. Anyway, as she told the nurse, if that doctor ever tried to give her pills, she'd flush them down the toilet.

YOUR EMOTIONS: A POWERFUL PULL

The first step in living well with diabetes is not going on a diet or taking pills. It's not insulin or finding the best doctor. The first step in taking care of your diabetes is *taking care of your emotions*. Diabetes is a serious and chronic illness, and the diagnosis stirs fear in many people. People think at once of shots and food deprivation, of being different, of losing limbs and going blind, or of dying young. No two ways about it, hearing you have diabetes is bad news.

When people hear bad news, it's normal for them to have a series of typical responses:

- Disbelief *("No way this could happen to me!")*

- Denial *("The doctor got it all wrong. I'm fine.")*

- Grief *("I miss not eating or drinking what I want. I miss my life. Things will never be the same.")*

- Anger *("It's just not fair! This is all your fault!")*

- Bargaining *("I promise I'll do better, I'll take care of myself, dear God, just make this go away.")*

- Acceptance *("So be it. So it is. It's okay. I can handle it.")*

These feelings may come one after the other, in stages, or they can be all jumbled together. They can also go away, only to pop up again when least expected. If you let your emotions get the better of you, it can be hazardous to your health. You might ignore the fact that you have diabetes, eating and drinking what you want until you get sick. You might feel too depressed to go outside, let alone exercise. You might feel so anxious that you can't even think of checking your sugar. You might be so angry that you won't see you doctor—or ask your family and friends for their support.

Only when you are able to deal with your emotions can you make the changes necessary to live well with diabetes. And to deal with your emotions you have to admit to them and to think about them. It might also help to discuss them with someone whose judgment you respect, whether that is a family member, a friend, a pastor, a mental health professional, or members of a support group.

Angela, in our example, was used to feeling in control of herself and her career. Finding out she had diabetes was a terrible shock to her because it made her feel like she was out of control.

Most people feel more than just one negative emotion when they learn that they have diabetes. Let's take a look at some of them, considering both why you might react in such a way and what you can do about it.

Shock

You might be in shock if:

- You feel numb.

- Your mind feels slow and stuck.

When someone hears he or she has a serious illness, it's normal for that person to go into shock. Shock is that dazed feeling that we get when something life-changing happens to us. Shock protects us for a little while by making us numb, which gives us time to adjust to the pile of other feelings about to come our way.

Denial

You might be in denial if you:

- Think that your blood sugar being just a little high means you don't really have diabetes.

- Think your diabetes is "mild" and that it can't cause you serious complications if left untreated.

- Decide there's no point in dealing with your diabetes because "everybody has to die sometime" and you'd rather enjoy life.

- Consider doing something you actually know is bad for you (like throwing away medications the doctor gives you).

- Postpone taking care of your health because you are "too busy."

Denial means refusing to believe something that is true and obvious. It is normally one of a person's first reactions to bad news. As long as denial remains just that—a first reaction—being in denial can temporarily be helpful by allowing us to digest all the new and unwelcome information more slowly. Angela, for example, wanted to believe that maybe she didn't have diabetes because the nurse told her that her diabetes was "mild." Even though Angela was smart enough to know that the tests proved she had diabetes, thinking about what that meant was so overwhelming she couldn't deal with it. The good news was that, while a part of Angela didn't believe she had diabetes, the other part was already taking steps to take care of herself by cutting down on desserts at the Christmas party.

Until Angela fully accepted that she had diabetes, she wouldn't take care of herself as well as she possibly could.

Isolation

You might be isolating yourself if you:

- Avoid people and situations.

- Think no one else can understand what you're going through.

Another common result of hearing bad health news is to think you are different from other people. You may feel that you are the only person in the world with your particular health problem, even though you know that a lot of people have diabetes. You may avoid people so you don't have to discuss your health with them. You may feel that it's too much trouble to try to function in the world given all the work you must do to take care of your condition.

Diabetes *will* change how you function in the world. You will be in a different situation than most other people. But you are not alone. Don't let yourself feel lonelier than you have to. You will have to plan ahead, create schedules, restrict your eating, schedule your medication, exercise, and plan doctor's appointments. If you try to hide all this from family and friends, you will lay a heavy additional burden on yourself. Angela was able to go to the Christmas party instead of avoiding it and becoming more isolated.

Certainly, people with diabetes, like everybody else, have a right to their privacy. Not everyone has to know everything about your health. But be careful that you're not lying because you are ashamed of yourself. Some people are embarrassed about their diabetes because they feel they brought it upon themselves. In fact, nobody is to blame for diabetes! Other people may not tell their families because they don't want them to worry. If you choose not to tell people about your diabetes (although this is not the strategy we recommend), be clear with yourself about *why* you made that choice.

Anger

You might be angry if you:

- Find yourself getting irritated a lot more.

- Are more easily offended and hurt.

- Have lots of tension in your face and neck.

It is not fair. Why you? Getting an illness is hard. Dealing with diabetes will take a chunk of your time, your emotional energy, and, possibly, your money—at least in the beginning. You may resent having to schedule your life around taking care of your diabetes. You may feel you have to deprive yourself of your favorite foods. You may get frustrated at figuring out medication doses and blood sugar levels. You will certainly believe that developing diabetes isn't fair.

When faced with difficulties, anger is a normal emotion. Since you can't really get angry at a disease, your anger might turn to the people around you. You may think your spouse is insensitive to keep eating dessert when you cannot. You may get annoyed with your doctor, who acts too rushed and doesn't answer your questions in a way you understand.

As with your other emotions, you will have better control if you can admit your anger to yourself. If you think about it, you can probably use the anger to your advantage. Instead of fuming about things, use your anger to identify problems you have to solve. Many specific sources of anger can be resolved that way. You can't get rid of diabetes, but you can talk with your spouse about supporting your eating habits. You can and should ask your doctor to take the time to answer all your questions completely.

Guilt

You might be feeling guilt if you:

- Think you are hurting other people if you take care of yourself.

- Blame yourself for getting diabetes.

It is not your fault. Diabetes sometimes feels as if it's going to turn your life upside down, and that's bound to have some affect on those around you. You may have to take time off from work to go to medical appointments. Maybe you need to spend your money on medicine instead of on a new toy for your child. It's important that you make your health a priority, even if that means not doing as much for those around you. Many people feel guilty about putting their own health first. In this society, we are used to running ourselves ragged with responsibilities and work. We often find it hard to cut back on both to take care of our health. And we often feel very guilty when we try.

Other people may feel guilty because they didn't overcome risk factors for diabetes. Remember, if you are overweight, you did not give yourself diabetes. And kicking yourself will not do any good. Some overweight people will never get diabetes, but many do. Think of it this way: If you've gotten diabetes, you've also gotten the signal to improve your lifestyle.

Sadness

You might be sad if you:

- Keep thinking about how much you've lost.

This is probably the most common response to bad news. Learning you have diabetes can take away the image of yourself as healthy. You may feel you have lost the life you had imagined for yourself (even though, eventually, it most likely won't turn out to be as bad as you imagine.) You may feel sad because you feel the diabetes makes you different from those around you. You may mourn the food you think you'll have to give up. You may miss your healthy, seemingly indestructible, old body.

Depression

You might be depressed if you:

- Cry too much—or too easily.

- Sleep too little—or sleep too much.

- Lack an appetite.

- Feel bad about yourself.

- Feel hopeless and helpless.

- Have no energy.

- Do not look forward to anything.

- Think about hurting yourself.

- Have aches and pains that aren't related to physical activities.

You may become depressed just thinking about your health. But most people feel better as they learn to care for themselves and get used to their diet, exercise, and medication regimen. However, if you find that your blues just won't go away, you should talk with your health care provider. Studies show that people with diabetes suffer from depression up to four times as much as the general public. Depression is a common reaction and there is no shame in it. What *is* a shame is to stay depressed when so many treatments are now available. Depression is a serious illness, and without treatment it will make it very difficult for you to care for your diabetes.

Most people feel better as they learn to care for themselves and get used to their diet, exercise, and medication regimen.

Fear

You might be fearful if you worry about:

- What the future holds for you.

- Uncomfortable shots and tests.

- Complications of diabetes.

There is a lot to fear in diabetes. Insulin shots, blindness, amputation, and early death are all things that could happen to someone with diabetes. It's normal to think about the "worst-case scenario." However, with recent medical advances, treatment for diabetes is better than ever, and will continue to improve. The scary health problems you may have heard about are not likely to happen to you if you take good care of yourself.

Use fear to motivate you to check your sugar levels, to keep your doctor appointments, and to make time to take the best possible care of yourself.

Anxiety

You may be anxious if:

- You can't sleep.

- Your thoughts are racing or you can't concentrate.

- You have one or more of the physical symptoms of anxiety: a racing heart beat, chest pain, sweating, feeling faint, feeling sick to your stomach, feeling as if you can't catch your breath.

- You feel jittery.

- Your anxiety keeps you from caring for yourself (for example, testing your blood glucose).

Anxiety is fear that never goes away. It is constant and intense. If you are anxious, you may become unable to think of anything other than how having diabetes can hurt you. Being anxious is exhausting. You can become so overwhelmed with anxiety that you are unable to take care of your diabetes or to function in other parts of your life.

Your emotions are real and normal, but they are like little children. They want your attention now! You should respect them and listen to them, but if you are going to live your best life with diabetes, you are going to have to get your emotions under control.

Anxiety can be a normal response to something as stressful as hearing that you have diabetes. However, if the anxiety is interfering with your ability to function or to feel good, consider getting help from your health care provider.

WISDOM TO ACCEPT, WISDOM TO CHANGE

Wisdom comes from experience. Having diabetes will give you many experiences, both bad *and* good. You will have the shock and disappointment of your diagnosis. But you will also have pride in what you have learned about the disease and in how well you are taking care of yourself.

Some people find it helpful to remember the Serenity Prayer: "God grant me the serenity to accept the things I cannot change, the courage to change the things I can, and the wisdom to know the difference." Your emotions are real and normal, but they are like little children. They want your attention now! You should respect them and listen to them, but if you are going to live your best life with diabetes, you are going to have to get your emotions under control.

ANGELA TRIES TO DEAL
WITH HER EMOTIONS

It took a while for Angela to get used to the idea that she had diabetes, but after several months it didn't seem such a big deal. She felt much better now that she was checking her glucose levels and improving her diet. After she told some of her co-workers about her diabetes, one of them joined her for a walk during almost every lunch hour. Angela was relieved that she had gotten control of the situation. She was proud of herself because it had been hard.

When she went to her next doctor's appointment, Angela was completely unprepared to find out that, despite her hard work, her sugar was higher than before. Her doctor started talking about medication again. Angela had tried really hard, and done pretty well, and she thought the doctor was blaming her for her high sugar. She went home feeling hopeless, mad at the doctor, and mad at herself for thinking she had diabetes beat.

Setbacks

In life, there are always setbacks. It's good to be mentally prepared for them. And just as things can get worse, they can also get better again. People are surprised to feel the return of a painful emotion they thought they had overcome. The emotions often return, but, like echoes, they are usually shorter and less intense.

That "return" of negativity can sometimes happen if you are reminded that you have a limitation (such as not being able to take off your shoes at the beach because you are taking care of your feet). If you face a medical setback, all the bad feelings you thought you had overcome after your diabetes diagnosis could return. You might feel the denial, the anger, the fear, and the other negative pulls all over again.

The more you learn to handle your emotions, the better you will be at dealing with them when they pop up again.

Why Bother?

Managing diabetes is a lot of work, and we haven't even gotten to your diet, exercising, or medication! Just dealing with the emotions can be exhausting. Why bother? Remember that just by reading this book you have taken a big step in taking care of yourself. You may want to write down a list of your own reasons to be healthy. Then, when it really does seem too hard, you can remember what the stakes are. Here are some positive emotional practices that have helped other people:

- Think of all the things you look forward to and list them. They might include visiting a friend, going to the movies, taking a trip, or watching your child graduate. You will need to be healthy to do those things.

- Think of those you love. You want to be well so you can spend time with them.

- Think of your children or grandchildren. You are a powerful role model for them. When you set an example of taking good care of your health, you will help them care for their own health for the rest of their lives.

- Remember: This is the only life you have. You have diabetes. You are going to have a great life *with* diabetes!

Happiness

You can have diabetes and be happy. You can have diabetes and still be healthier than many people who don't have diabetes. If you follow the recommendations for eating, exercising, and managing your blood glucose, you will be doing more for your health than many other people out there. Yes, when you are first diagnosed you may feel that you have been dealt a terrible blow. Yes, it will take some adjusting to the reality of diabetes before you can feel normal again. But, yes, you *will* feel normal again.

Studies have researched the elements that may help people with diabetes be happy. These are the things you should look out for:

- *People with diabetes are happier when they exercise regularly.* We have already mentioned the importance of exercise in diabetes, and will go into it in more detail in Chapter Five.

- *Family support* helps people with diabetes feel more comfortable and at ease.

- *Good glucose control* is associated with a positive feeling of good health, even when insulin is necessary to achieve that control.

- *Give it time.* Most people with diabetes feel better about themselves as they get older and get used to living with diabetes.

- *Cultivating a good attitude* helps reinforce positive emotions. Every day, count the things for which you are thankful. Try to see what is funny in a situation. A sense of humor goes a long way.

- *Faith.* It may help you to draw on your faith in God.

- *Finding a good support group* gives a real sense of community. You are not alone. Talking with other people who are going through the same things as you, discovering insights, hints, and tips your healthcare provider and diabetes educators might not know, realizing that these people, who live with diabetes every day just like you, really know what it's like and really understand— these benefits are invaluable. The American Diabetes Association has lists of support groups in your area. Call 1–800–DIABETES (342–2383), visit *www.diabetes.org*, or contact your local hospital for more information.

ANGELA GOES HOME FOR THE HOLIDAYS

Angela planned her trip to her parent's house in New York carefully. She packed her medications in her carry-on luggage and called the airline ahead of time to order a diabetic meal. She also brought a snack with her in case the flight was delayed during take-off or it took too long before they served the meal.

Ever since Angela told her family about her diabetes, her mother took care to prepare food that Angela could eat. But the holidays offered a real challenge. Angela felt sad when her Aunt Sheila proudly offered a piece of her special Christmas rum cake. Everyone knew that Aunt Sheila fussed over that cake for weeks. But Angela had prepared herself emotionally. She knew not to feel guilty. She told Aunt Sheila how much she had loved the cake in the past, and accepted a tiny taste, but she passed on the big slice that Aunt Sheila was offering. She thought back on all the good memories she had with her family and thought of how they'd have fun in the future. Rum cake wasn't the only route to happiness!

Dealing with Your Friends and Family

Your relationships with the people in your life have a big impact on your happiness. When you learn you have diabetes, those relationships may change. Some people might seem unsupportive of your attempts to improve your lifestyle. Others might be overbearing and smother you with their advice. Yet others may surprise you with their thoughtfulness.

It's your choice how much to tell other people about your diabetes. It's probably a good idea to tell a few close friends, and some people at work, in case of emergencies. Remember there is no shame in having diabetes. It is a very common health problem; chances are that you are not the only person in the room with it. If you tell other people that you have diabetes, they will be better able to support you in your daily choices to eat right and exercise.

Meals

Sometimes people get very emotional about food. Besides nourishment, food has a lot of meaning in our culture. Food helps us celebrate, it helps us honor traditions, and it comforts us. Even though you have diabetes, other people may become upset when you don't eat their food.

Try to be polite, but firm. If someone insists you eat something you know isn't good for you, tell her you have diabetes and can't eat it. You can tell her you'll take it home to have later (and give it to someone at home). Or you can have a tiny piece. In the next chapter, we'll discuss diet, one of the key elements for diabetes treatment.

Exercise

Exercise with your friends or with family members. Exercise benefits almost everybody and it's a fun activity you can share. (We'll give you some ideas in Chapter Six.)

Remember:

- It's normal to be upset about a diagnosis of diabetes.

- Don't deny your feelings; most people feel better with time.

- Get help if you feel overwhelmed.

- The more your family knows about diabetes, the more helpful they can be.

CHAPTER FIVE

EATING SMART

SHEILA STRESSES OUT

When Sheila found out that she had type 2 diabetes, her first thought was that she'd have to give up food. Sheila loved food, and she had the full figure to prove it. She had tried to lose weight several times and dreaded having to deprive herself again, having to count calories and eat weird, bland food. She had heard about people with diabetes carrying little books around and checking everything they ate and weighing their food, and it just seemed like more trouble than she'd ever be able to take on, let alone keep up.

The day before her appointment with her dietician, Sheila went home and ate a pizza and a pint of ice cream, figuring it would be her last. She felt terrible afterwards. So, she was pleasantly surprised (and a little skeptical) when she met with the dietician, who told her that she didn't have to begin a strict diet. However, the dietician did want Shelia to count calories so that she could lose weight. They planned on talking the following week to discuss Shelia's progress.

CHANGING YOUR EATING BEHAVIOR

In one way, you are fortunate. Your diagnosis of diabetes is prompting you to eat healthily. The diet we recommend is advisable for everyone, not just for people with diabetes. If you make the changes we recommend in the way you eat and in what you eat, you will not only improve your blood sugar, but also lower your risk of heart disease—which is also a high risk for all Americans. You will also become a powerful role model by eating a healthy diet. The lifestyle improvements you set in motion will go on to benefit your children's attitudes and health.

We live in the land of "bigger is better," super-sized meals, all-you-can-eat buffets, and fast food. In today's world, many of us feel too busy to fix dinner every evening. Instead, we sit in front of our televisions, bombarded by advertisements for food and weight-loss plans. The food that is advertised is generally overly-processed and high in salt, sugar and fat, but low in nutrition. The weight-loss plans are expensive and may often be ineffective or even dangerous.

THE DASH EATING PLAN

No, this has nothing to do with eating fast. DASH is short for a study called Dietary Approaches to Stop Hypertension. DASH found that the risk of elevated blood pressure could be reduced with a low-fat eating plan that is rich in low-fat foods, dairy foods, fruits, and vegetables. The plan is rich in calcium, potassium, and magnesium. It has also been found to be ideal for people with diabetes because it keeps blood sugar on an even keel.

THE DASH DIET
BASED ON 2000 CALORIES PER DAY

Food Group	Daily Servings	Serving Size	Examples and Notes
Grains and grain products	7–8	· 1 slice bread · ½ cup dry cereal · ½ cup cooked rice, pasta, or cereal	whole wheat bread, English muffin, pita bread, bagel, cereals, grits, oatmeal
Vegetables	4–5	· 1 cup raw leafy vegetable · ½ cup cooked vegetable · 6 oz. vegetable juice	tomatoes, potatoes, carrots, peas, squash, broccoli, turnip greens, collards, kale, spinach, artichokes, beans, sweet potatoes
Fruits	4–5	· 6 oz. fruit juice · 1 medium fruit · ¼ cup dried fruit · ½ cup fresh, frozen, or canned fruit	apricots, bananas, dates, grapes, oranges, orange juice, grapefruit, grapefruit juice, melons, mangoes, peaches, pineapples, prunes, raisins, strawberries, tangerines
Low-fat or nonfat dairy	2–3	· 8 oz. milk · 1 cup yogurt · 1½ oz. cheese	skim or 1% milk, skim or low-fat buttermilk, nonfat or low-fat yogurt, part skim mozzarella cheese, nonfat cheese
Meats, poultry, and fish	2	3 oz. cooked meats, poultry, or fish	lean meats (trimmed of visible fat), broiled, roasted or baked poultry with skin removed

Food Group	Daily Servings	Serving Size	Examples and Notes
Nuts, seeds, and legumes	4–5 per week	· 1½ oz. or ¼ cup nuts · ½ oz. or 2 Tbsp. seeds · ½ cup cooked legumes	almonds, filberts, mixed nuts, peanuts, walnuts, sunflower seeds, kidney beans, lentils

DASH MEAL PLAN SUGGESTIONS BASED ON 1500 CALORIES PER DAY

Food	Servings Amount	Provides
Breakfast		
orange juice	6 ounces	1 fruit
skim milk	8 ounces (1 cup)	1 dairy
corn flakes (with 1 t sugar)	¾ cup	1½ grains
banana	1 medium	1 fruit
lite whole wheat bread (with 1 T jelly)	1 slice	1 grain
Lunch		
baked chicken	3 ounces	1 poultry
pita bread	½ slice, large	1 grain
raw vegetable medley:		
carrot & celery sticks	3–4 sticks each	1 vegetable
radishes	2	
loose-leaf lettuce	2 leaves	
part skim mozzarella cheese	1½ slices (1½ ounces)	1 dairy
skim milk	8 ounces	1 dairy
fruit cocktail in water	½ cup	1 fruit
Dinner		
herbed baked cod	3 ounces	1 fish
scallion rice	½ cup	1 grain
steamed broccoli	½ cup	1 vegetable
stewed tomatoes	½ cup	1 vegetable
spinach salad:		
raw spinach	½ cup	1 vegetable
cherry tomatoes	2	
cucumber	2 slices	
lite Italian salad dressing	1 tablespoon	½ fat

EATING SMART

Food	Servings Amount	Provides
soft margarine	1 teaspoon	1 fat
melon balls	½ cup	1 fruit

Snacks

mini-pretzels	1 ounce (¾ cup)	1 grain
mixed nuts	2 tablespoons	¾ nuts
diet ginger ale	12 ounces	0

Total number of servings in this 1500 calories per day menu:

Food Group	Servings
Grains	5.5
Vegetables	4
Fruits	4
Dairy Foods	3
Meats, Poultry, Fish	2
Nuts	¾
Fats & Oils	1½

Tips on eating the DASH way:

· Start small. Make gradual changes in your eating habits.
· Center your meal around carbohydrates, such as pasta, rice, beans, or vegetables.
· Treat meat as one part of the whole meal, instead of the focus.
· Use fruits or low-fat, low-calorie foods such as sugar-free gelatin for desserts and snacks.

REMEMBER! If you use the DASH diet to help prevent or control high blood pressure, make it part of a lifestyle that includes choosing foods lower in salt and sodium, keeping a healthy weight, being physically active, and, if you drink alcohol, doing so in moderation.

Sources: Zernel, M. B. (1997), Dietary Patterns and Hypertension: The DASH Study. *Nutrition Review*, 55: 303–305. Developed with assistance from Annette Cole, UIUC Graduate Dietetic Intern

Additional DASH information is available from the following web sites: National Institute of Health—http://www.nhlbi.nih.gov/health/public/heart/hbp/dash/index.htm

LOSE THE EXTRA WEIGHT

If you are overweight, you do need to lose the extra pounds. By losing weight, your diabetes will improve, and it may even go away. The people in the Diabetes Prevention Program (*see Chapter Two*) were able to ward off diabetes by losing an average of just 10 pounds. Furthermore, losing weight will decrease your chance of having high blood pressure and high cholesterol, conditions that often afflict people with diabetes.

Even if you don't need to lose weight, you should exercise portion control. Eat more healthy food. Avoid fast food and prepared foods. Start reading food labels (*see page 50*). As you continue to eat healthier foods, your taste buds will learn to do without so much sugar, salt, and fat.

Healthy diet is a subject about which we have *too much* information. Unfortunately, much of the information is confusing, conflicting, and controversial. Different people recommend different strategies for eating: fat free, low carb, exchange lists, pyramids, and even glycemic indexes. One of these may be right for you, but buyer beware. There are lots of companies trying to sell you diets and miracle supplements.

In our view, the way to eat a healthy diet is no secret. In the context of diabetes, it's even more essential because if you don't, you risking getting the disease. Our ancestors didn't have as much diabetes—they weren't on the latest fad diet.

The rules for eating well are simple. We'll spend the rest of the chapter discussing them.

Rules of Healthy Eating

- Remember what, when, why, where, and how.

- Eat at the table.

- Portion size is key.

- Never "super-size" it.

- Plan ahead.

- Don't skip meals.

- Less processed is better.

- Trade less healthy foods for more healthy foods.

- Eat something green with lunch and dinner.

- Learn to prepare foods in a healthier way.[1]

- Avoid food that is bad for you.

- Remember: You can eat anything, but you can't eat *everything*

What, When, Why, Where and How?

We eat to live, to celebrate, to comfort ourselves, and to express our culture. What we eat and how we eat help define our identity. No wonder people feel very concerned about having to change their diets. However, if you have diabetes, you'd better take a close look at how you eat. Chances are your health will benefit.

Eating right involves paying attention not just to what you eat, but also to *why* you eat it. If you eat every time you're stressed

---

1. For a list of heart healthy recipes, see the appendix, as well as visiting www.hiltonpub.com and reading, *The Heart of the Matter* by Hilton M. Hudson, M.D., F.A.C.S. (Rockford, IL: Hilton Publishing, 2000.)

out, you will gain weight and be less healthy—even if you eat really healthy food. If you eat in front of the TV, chances are you won't notice your stomach's signals that you've eaten enough— and you'll eat more than you need.

What should you eat? Healthy food. (You'll read more about this later on in this chapter.)

When should you eat? At least three times a day. Many experts recommend adding small snacks. The point is not to let yourself get so hungry that you might overeat.

Why should you eat? To stay healthy, because it's mealtime, because you're hungry.

Why should you *not* eat? Because you are upset or bored. Neither should you eat just to please other people.

Where should you eat? At the table. A meal is an event and a ritual. The more special you make your meal (think nice napkins, dishes, perhaps candles) the more satisfied you will feel. If you eat standing in front of the refrigerator, while driving, or while watching the TV news, you won't feel as satisfied. Under such circumstances, you are likely to eat more and enjoy it less.

How should you eat? By paying attention to your food. Take your time; enjoy the flavors. The more attention you give your food, the more you will enjoy it, and the more satisfied you will feel. Eat slowly. This gives your stomach time to signal your brain that you're full. Stop eating when you first start to feel full. Don't feel that you have to finish off your plate.

Portion Size is Key

Whether you are trying to lose weight or just to keep your sugar stable, you must limit the amount of what you eat. Our culture makes this hard. Everything seems to be getting bigger: cookies, steaks, and cans of soda. The result is bigger people with more diabetes and more heart disease. Our bodies are designed to avoid starvation; in times of plenty, we store fat. Centuries ago when we were hunters, gatherers, and farmers, famine was a way of life. Today, most of us in the United States have too much food—all the time.

Read Your Labels

The "Nutrition Facts" label printed on every food package is so common a sight, you usually don't even notice it. But it holds a vital key to your health. Reading the labels on all your foods can make the difference between eating well and undermining your good health.

Governmental rules require each label to report specific items. At the top of every list, you will find the serving size and the number of servings per container. You might be surprised to see that what you thought was one portion is actually two-and-a-half portions! If you hadn't checked the label, you'd be eating two-and-a-half times more than you thought you were. The label also provides helpful nutritional information, such as how many calories there are in a serving, as well as the amount of fat, sodium, and carbohydrates in each. The list of ingredients usu-ally follows below this information (*See illustration, page 62*).

You also need to have an idea of what an ounce or cupful looks like. Pull out your measuring cups and look at them. These comparisons can help:

Portion Size	About as big as
3 ounces of meat	A deck of cards
1 cup of juice or rice	A tennis ball

FOOD LABEL GUIDE

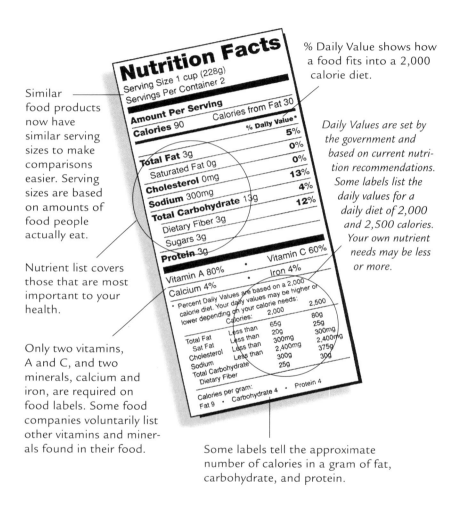

% Daily Value shows how a food fits into a 2,000 calorie diet.

Daily Values are set by the government and based on current nutrition recommendations. Some labels list the daily values for a daily diet of 2,000 and 2,500 calories. Your own nutrient needs may be less or more.

Similar food products now have similar serving sizes to make comparisons easier. Serving sizes are based on amounts of food people actually eat.

Nutrient list covers those that are most important to your health.

Only two vitamins, A and C, and two minerals, calcium and iron, are required on food labels. Some food companies voluntarily list other vitamins and minerals found in their food.

Some labels tell the approximate number of calories in a gram of fat, carbohydrate, and protein.

Nutrition Facts

Serving Size 1 cup (228g)
Servings Per Container 2

Amount Per Serving

Calories 90   Calories from Fat 30

% Daily Value *

Total Fat 3g   5%
Saturated Fat 0g   0%
Cholesterol 0mg   0%
Sodium 300mg   13%
Total Carbohydrate 13g   4%
Dietary Fiber 3g   12%
Sugars 3g
Protein 3g

Vitamin A 80%   •   Vitamin C 60%
Calcium 4%   •   Iron 4%

* Percent Daily Values are based on a 2,000 calorie diet. Your daily values may be higher or lower depending on your calorie needs:

		Calories:	2,000	2,500
Total Fat	Less than		65g	80g
Sat Fat	Less than		20g	25g
Cholesterol	Less than		300mg	300mg
Sodium	Less than		2,400mg	2,400mg
Total Carbohydrate			300g	375g
Dietary Fiber			25g	30g

Calories per gram:
Fat 9   •   Carbohydrate 4   •   Protein 4

Note: Numbers on nutrition labels may be rounded.

Don't make overeating easy. Keep serving platters off the table. Serve yourself, keeping portion size in mind, and eat sitting down. Eat slowly and pay attention to all the flavors in the food. Drink plenty of water.

Never Super-size It

Don't order the biggest sizes. Restaurants make the biggest sizes seem like a bargain, but they aren't. You probably don't need that much food, and having health complications is no bargain! If the portions you are served are too large, share the meal with your dining companion. Bring leftovers home. Remember that you don't have to clean off your plate!

SHEILA CHECKS IN

After a week, Sheila was eager to talk to the dietician. She had a lot of questions. For one thing, she was a busy woman and didn't really have time to cook things from scratch. Besides, she didn't know which packaged foods were healthy and which ones weren't. She also ate fast food at lunch because she didn't have the time or the money to sit down in a restaurant. The dietician's advice had sounded pretty simple, but it wasn't realistic.

When Sheila told her about these difficulties, the dietician gave her some strategies. She told Sheila to:

1. *Read the nutrition labels that come on all packaged food so she could learn the nutritional content of food.*
2. *Plan meals ahead of time. For meals at home, she advised Sheila to cook several batches of food at a time and freeze them for later use. Sheila was surprised to hear how many cookbooks were available for people with diabetes. She didn't*

know that Patti LaBelle had just written one, and planned to stop by the library to check it out.

3. *Pack her own lunch a few days a week. If Sheila wanted to eat in fast food restaurants, she should order grilled chicken or fish (not fried). She should avoid hamburgers, anything fried, and desserts. She should get acquainted with the salad bar, but be careful about some of the toppings and side dishes, such as bacon bits or macaroni salad. And she should choose the oil and vinegar dressing; it's the healthiest and lowest in calories. The dietician also gave Sheila a booklet that listed the caloric content of different types of fast food.[1]*

Sheila realized she could eat healthier if she worked at it. She kind of resented having to work at eating, but she wanted to feel better—so she planned to give it a shot.

PLAN AHEAD

To control your diet, you need to plan ahead. Don't be caught starving at mealtime and not knowing what to eat. If you're on medication for diabetes, being unprepared could lead to hypoglycemia, a potentially dangerous condition in which your sugar goes too low (*see Chapter Seven*). On a less serious note, being unprepared can also narrow your food choices. If you don't plan ahead, you have to eat whatever you can get—and this is most likely not going to be the healthiest thing for you.

At first, you may need extra time and planning to prepare your

---

1. Call the American Diabetes Association at 1–800–DIABETES or visit their web site, www.diabetes.org for information on fast foods.

meals; you will need time to familiarize yourself with the foods that are the best for you—as well as ways to prepare them so that they are most tasty. As you get used to planning in advance, you'll need less time and thought to plan, but you should still have a good idea of what your next meal will be beforehand.

Planning ahead allows you to buy food in advance. You can stock up on the healthy foods we list below. That way you won't be stuck having to buy whatever is in a fast food restaurant or vending machine. Not only is it healthier to plan ahead, it's cheaper!

If you do end up eating at a fast food restaurant, you can still be prepared. Many fast food restaurants now list the nutritional content of their food. Ask to see the list. You can also purchase small pocket guides to restaurant food so that you'll know which choices are the healthiest.

Planning ahead can also mean cooking meals ahead of time and freezing them for later use. This way, if you are too tired to cook, you just defrost your meal.

Stock your kitchen with the following healthy—and fast—food:

- Frozen lean cuts of meat

- Frozen vegetables

- Whole grain pasta

- Canned beans (check for salt content)

- Apples

- Oranges

- Pre-washed carrot sticks

- Unsalted nuts

- Plain low-fat yogurt

- Salad in a bag

- Certain frozen meals, if the label shows they're healthy

With these supplies, a microwave, and a stove, you can have dinner whipped up within half an hour.

DON'T SKIP MEALS

A lot of people skip breakfast. Unfortunately, if you skip breakfast, you may end up hungry in the middle of the morning or starving by lunch. Eat a light meal before you get too hungry. It's best to eat at the table, but if you really can't, bring a snack with you. If you get too hungry, you're more likely to overeat, more likely to eat something unhealthy—and at a greater risk for hypoglycemia to boot.

LESS PROCESSED IS BETTER

We all get more sugar, salt, and fat than we need. This is especially true if you have diabetes. Obviously, if you have diabetes you want to minimize added sugar. Most people with type 2 diabetes are overweight and also need to minimize fats, since they are high in calories and cause us to gain weight. And, since most people with type 2 diabetes are prone to high blood pressure, they will also need to minimize salt.

One of the easiest ways to avoid salt, fat, and sugar is to stop buying processed foods.

Processed foods are foods that have been prepared in a factory. They generally contain more salt, sugar, fat, and preservatives to keep their taste fresh. Some examples are canned soups, sweet juice drinks, cold cuts, and frozen meals. When you eat processed foods, you are getting less of the food itself and more of the additives. Check the label carefully before you purchase a frozen dinner.

We all get more sugar, salt, and fat than we need. This is especially true if you have diabetes.

Many processed food companies are trying to appeal to our desire to eat more healthfully, and you may be able to find frozen meals, canned foods, and juice drinks without all the additives. Some fast food companies are also featuring more healthy foods and portions.

Thus, it's better to buy meat and cook it than to buy the cold cuts. It's much healthier to eat a piece of fruit than to drink a fruit drink. And it's generally healthier to cook a meal than to buy a frozen dinner.

A different category of processing applies to complex carbohydrate foods such as wheat and rice. These grains are originally brown, but are often processed to create white rice and white wheat for white bread. Whole wheat and brown rice are much better for your blood sugar than their white counterparts.

TRADE LESS HEALTHY FOR MORE HEALTHY FOODS

Meet with your dietician to learn all you can about healthy eating. She'll help you to understand, and plan for a healthy diet. Here in the box below are the basic principles of what she'll tell you.

BETTER CHOICES FOR A HEALTHY LIFESTYLE

Decrease	Increase
Simple carbohydrates	**Complex carbohydrates**
Corn flakes	Bran cereal, oatmeal
White bread	Whole wheat bread
Potatoes	Green leafy vegetables
French fries	Broccoli, cabbage
Corn	Beans
White rice	Brown rice
Pasta	Whole wheat pasta
Fruit juice	Piece of fresh fruit
Fatty meats	**Lean meats, or, better yet, fish or soy**
Beef	Lean beef
Ground beef	Ground turkey
Bacon	Smoked turkey
Fried chicken	Grilled chicken
Hamburger	Grilled chicken or veggie sandwich
Bottled dressing	Oil, vinegar, and herbs
Snacks	**Healthy snacks**
Corn chips	Carrot sticks
Potato chips	Pretzels
Donut	Whole wheat bagel
Candy bar	Piece of fresh fruit
Soda	Diet soda, water (with or without lemon)
Fried foods	Grilled, broiled, baked foods
Lard, butter, margarine	Olive oil
Whole dairy products	**Low-fat dairy products**
Condiments	**Healthy condiments**
Salt	Herbs and spices, lemon, garlic
Sugar	Artificial sweetener
	High fructose corn syrup

To stabilize our blood sugar and protect our hearts, experts generally agree that we should eat more:

- Green vegetables.

- Beans, more accurately called *legumes*. These include black beans, pinto beans, and lentils. (Green beans are great, but they are vegetables and not in this category.)

- Fish, especially fish high in omega-3 fatty acids, such as salmon and sardines.

- Nuts. (Be careful with portion size—nuts are high in calories. And make sure to eat nuts with no added salt.)

- Fiber: fruit, vegetables, whole grains, and beans are all high in fiber.

Start buying more of these items. Learn to prepare them to your liking, and make them the mainstay of your diet.

Eat Something Green with Lunch and Dinner

Green vegetables, like collards, broccoli, peppers, and spinach, for example, are very healthy. They are high in fiber, which can lower your cholesterol and your sugar, and may also lower your risk of cancer. They are high in a variety of vitamins. And no, you can't take a fiber pill and a vitamin pill instead. The health benefits are not the same. Groceries are now making your job easier by packaging pre-cut and pre-washed vegetables to minimize the work of preparing them. Experiment and find green vegetables you like and eat them at least twice a day. If you don't like any greens, find a cookbook on diabetes and read through it. You're sure to be inspired!

Learn to Prepare Foods in a Healthier Way

Jambalaya, pork roast, sweet potatoes, and apple crisp. Sounds good? Believe it or not, this is what you could be eating—if you learn to prepare them in a healthy way. You'll find these and other delicious recipes in *New Soul Food Cookbook for People with Diabetes* by Fabiola Demps Gaines and Roneice Weaver (McGraw-Hill/Contemporary Distributed Products, 1998) and *The Heart of the Matter,* by Hilton M. Hudson, M.D. and Herbert Stern, Ph.D. (Hilton Publishing Company, 2000) and in a variety of cookbooks published by the American Diabetes Association. (See the appendix for some of these great-tasting recipes) There are also many excellent cookbooks written specifically for African-American people with diabetes. Let diabetes prompt you to enjoy a healthier *and* tastier diet.

SHEILA SEES AN OLD FRIEND

A few months after she started dieting, Sheila saw a familiar face while she was at the supermarket buying her groceries for the week. It was her dietician. Sheila rushed over to say, "Hi, remember me? I'm Sheila! You helped me so much and I never did thank you." The dietician smiled at Sheila, "Oh, I remember you. Back then, you were too busy to shop." Sheila waved a bag of broccoli at her. "I'm eating my vegetables and loving them. My sugar levels are great, and I lost eight pounds!" Sheila walked off feeling happy. She really did feel much better since she had learned to eat healthy food.

Avoid Food that is Bad For You

Start by avoiding fried food, sweets, soda and other sugary drinks, fatty meats, and salty snack food. Replace unhealthy food with healthy food. Don't keep unhealthy food in the house. There's no need to tempt fate—or yourself. And don't feel sorry for the rest of the family. Your new diet is good for them as well.

Limit Your Alcohol Intake

Alcohol is high in carbohydrates, which can rapidly raise your blood sugar. It has little nutritional value. Alcohol can also precipitate hypoglycemia. It can cloud your judgment and lead to liver disease. Despite these dangers, scientists do believe a moderate amount of alcohol may have some health benefits. So if you do choose to drink, limit yourself to no more than one ounce per day.

SHEILA KICKS HERSELF

Sheila was so upset. After an unpleasant argument with a co-worker, Sheila had stopped at a convenience store on the way home. She bought a gallon of ice cream and finished it off as soon as she walked in her front door. She felt horrible afterward. The cheap ice cream had left a bad taste in her mouth, and she dreaded to check her blood glucose.

Sheila pulled out the dietician's business card the next day and gave her a call. The dietician told her that many people eat sweets like ice cream or chocolate when they are upset. She advised Sheila to think of alternative ways to deal with stress. Then she surprised Sheila by telling her that if she really wanted ice cream on occasion, she should get it—but it should be her favorite kind. She should try to eat just one cup, scooped into a pretty bowl while sitting at her table. She told Sheila to eat the ice cream slowly and to savor every bite.

You Can Eat Anything, But You Can't Eat Everything

The good news about eating when you have diabetes is that nothing is 100 percent off limits. For example, doctors used to tell their patients that they couldn't eat anything with sugar in it. Now we know that we don't need to be that restrictive. You should avoid sugar whenever you can, but if, on occasion, you want something sweet you can take steps to protect yourself. Eat just a little bit. (Less than a portion size.) Monitor your blood sugar afterwards and cut back on other complex carbohydrates. If you have a sweet tooth, get to know the many available artificial sweeteners.

If you've stuck to a healthy diet all week and you would just love some French fries, have some. But again, don't eat too many, and stick to healthy foods for the rest of the day. And when you do treat yourself, make sure it's something you really love.

Remember

- Lose weight if you are overweight.

- Keep portion size in mind.

- Plan your meals ahead of time.

- Eat more green vegetables, fruits, beans, whole grains, nonfat dairy products, and fish.

- Eat less processed foods, fried foods, meats, and sweets.

CHAPTER SIX

GET MOVING!

CHARLENE DOESN'T BUDGE

Charlene had been diagnosed with diabetes about a year ago. Her sugars were okay, but not good enough for her doctor. She was on a high dose of medication and she was following her diet pretty well—but she wasn't exercising. Her doctor kept nagging her to become more active, but Charlene hated exercise. She felt it was undignified. She didn't want to wear tight clothes and she didn't want to sweat. She paid good money to her hairdresser every two weeks. She had no intention of messing up her hairstyle. She asked the doctor if there wasn't some other medication she could take.

Exercise is a crucial part of treating your diabetes and living your best life. Exercise doesn't necessarily mean doing aerobics or lifting weights. It can be any kind of physical activity that gets you moving.

Americans in general have become fat and out of shape. We even tend to be fatter than the people still living in the countries

A SMALL MOVE–A BIG RESULT

Research has shown that just by walking half an hour a day, people can improve their health dramatically. When the participants of the Diabetes Prevention Program walked half an hour a day, five days a week, and in addition, began to eat a healthier diet, they lost an average of ten pounds and reduced their risk of diabetes by 60 percent! Simple lifestyle changes can have a big impact on your health.

of our ancestors. When early generations arrived in this country, most of them had to do hard physical work. Being sedentary was a privilege few could enjoy. It is only in the past few decades, with the arrival of technologies that have made our lives easier, that we have become *mainly sedentary*. This literally means that we sit all day. Many of our communities are based on the car as the main mode of transportation. Walking used to be a natural part of life. We used to walk to work, to visit other people, and to get to public transportation. Now we've totally changed our lifestyles. Think about it: if you commute to a desk job and watch TV in the evening, you are pretty much sitting all day. Your body was made to do more than that.

Now that physical activity is not naturally integrated into our lives, we consciously have to make room for it. Remember, we are moving to be healthier and happier. This is not a competition. This is not the time to be self-conscious about your appearance or your skill. You are doing this for yourself. You don't have to be the best, or even good. You just have to get moving. Eventually, it will become a good habit.

Exercise helps your diabetes in several ways:

Benefits of exercise

By exercising you can:

- Reverse insulin resistance.

- Help control weight.

- Lower blood pressure.

- Lower risk of heart disease.

- Decrease "bad" cholesterol (LDL) and increase "good" cholesterol (HDL).

- Help stress management.

- Improve quality of life.

- Build muscle.

Exercise Decreases Insulin Resistance

The main problem in type 2 diabetes is that your tissues are resistant to insulin. Exercise helps lower that resistance by sensitizing your cells to insulin. When you exercise, your muscles need glucose to burn as fuel. Since insulin helps cells absorb glucose, your "hungry" muscles become more sensitive to it—so they can get the glucose they need. This sensitivity begins soon after you start exercising and can last for up to twelve hours. If you check your blood glucose, you will notice that it is lower during this period of time. You may require less insulin or medication—or you may be able to stop taking medication all together!

Exercise is a Key Part of a Weight-Loss Program

When we exercise, we use calories that might otherwise go into fat production. This helps us lose weight, especially when combined with a lower calorie diet. Because obesity is a major cause of type 2 diabetes, weight loss through exercise can lead to better glucose control. And the benefits of exercise keep on going. Exercise not only burns calories while you work out, it also raises your metabolism, so you burn more calories afterwards.

Exercise Lowers Your Risk of Heart Disease

Apart from its effect on your diabetes control, exercise can reduce your risk of heart disease. Along with diabetes, hypertension (high blood pressure) and high cholesterol are major risk factors for heart disease. People who exercise have a reduced risk of hypertension, a major disease among African Americans. Moderate exercise lowers your blood pressure. In addition, physical activity can help reduce your "bad" cholesterol, a fatty substance that can clog your arteries.

Exercise is a Wonderful Way to Reduce Stress

The pressures, conflicts, and problems we live with in this society cause most daily stress. When we find ourselves in stressful situations, our body puts out hormones originally designed to help us fight an enemy or flee a danger. These are known as "fight or flight" hormones. These hormones are what make you get sweaty or dizzy when you are very upset. But these hormones not only make us feel bad; they can actually make us sick. A host of medical problems, such as heart disease, cancer, asthma, hypertension, and depression have been linked to stress. Studies have shown that exercise can reduce these stress hormones.

Exercise Improves Our Quality of Life

In addition to all the ways in which exercise helps our health, it just plain feels good. Exercise releases endorphins, hormones that lift our spirits naturally. After exercising many people feel a "natural high." But don't worry, it's legal, it's healthy, and it's nonfattening!

Besides all this, exercise offers these additional benefits:

- Stronger muscles.

- Stronger bones.

- More energy.

- More restful sleep.

- Better attitude.

- Better able to meet new people.

Now if someone offered you a medication that could do all that, wouldn't you buy it? But exercise is all-natural and it's free.

HOW TO START

Convinced? How do you start exercising? If you haven't moved much in a while, you are safer starting out slowly to reduce your risk of injury. Your goal is to exercise at a moderate level for half an hour a day, five days a week. This is how the participants of the Diabetes Prevention Program lost weight and improved their health. They walked at a pace fast enough to get their heart rates up, but slow enough so that they can still talk to one another.

It's *always* a good idea to discuss your exercise plans with your doctor. But please don't let this precaution be an excuse to delay your getting in shape. Phone your doctor today!

What should you do? Exercise doesn't have to be something formal; you don't have to wear a special outfit or belong to a gym. It can be something as simple as getting off the bus a few stops too soon every day and walking the extra distance home or to work. It can be putting the remote control away, and getting up during commercials and walking around the house.

As long as you get moving, and you do it safely, you are free to use your imagination. Do whatever you want! Don't be afraid to try a new sport. If you fear being "bad" at something, don't worry. Your only comparison should be with yourself. This is

---

SOME OTHER IDEAS TO GET YOU MOVING

· Walk around the block or around the mall.

· Swim.

· Dance.

· Take the stairs.

· Get a dog and take him for walks.

· Go bowling.

· Table tennis anyone?

· Clean your house.

· Garden.

exercising for good health and relaxation. Remember, this is not a competition. If you happen to enjoy competition, that's a fine reason to get exercise, too.

GETTING STARTED

If you are out of shape, you should start exercising gradually. Start your activity slowly and gradually pick up the pace. As you get into better shape, you can do it longer and harder.

Stretching

Stretching is an important part of your exercise regimen. Stretching warms your muscles up to minimize soreness and injuries. Move slowly until you feel the muscle stretch. It should feel relaxing. Hold the position for the count of twenty. Don't bounce. Breathe normally. Repeat the stretch about three times. Do this before and after your work out. It will help you feel limber and relaxed.

To avoid injuries, *warm up* and *cool down* before you stretch; just do your exercise less intensely at the beginning of your workout and at the end. For example, if you walk for exercise, you would walk less briskly for the first and last five minutes.

Other Tips

Slow down if you get out of breath. You should be able to talk while exercising without gasping for breath.

Drink lots of water before, during, and after exercise (even water workouts) to replace the water you lose by sweating.

STOP EXERCISING RIGHT AWAY IF YOU:

· Have any discomfort in your chest, neck, shoulder, or arm

· Feel dizzy or sick

· Break out in a cold sweat

· Have muscle cramps or pain in your joints, feet, ankles, or legs

Ask your health care provider what to do if you have any of these symptoms.

Keys to Success

Do something you enjoy. Exercise shouldn't be a chore. If you actually enjoy what you are doing, you are more likely to stick with it. You'll also be happier. If you dread the thought of exercise, try thinking about something you used to enjoy as a child. What about something you've always dreamed of doing? This is your chance. You may be surprised to discover that once you start moving, you'll fall in love with it. Remember, exercise releases endorphins, those feel-good hormones. Many people feel so good when they exercise that it becomes a favorite part of their day.

Exercise with a partner. Exercising with a partner is beneficial for three reasons. First, if you schedule an activity with someone, you are less likely to miss it. Second, if you're not wild about exercising, the social component of working out with a friend may be enough to make you enjoy the activity. Finally, if you feel unsafe walking by yourself, or if you feel self-conscious, say, about how you look in a bathing suit, going with a friend may give you the security and moral support you need. Of course, some people use exercise to think deeply or to daydream. And they prefer to be by themselves. Find what works best for you.

Incorporate exercise into your daily activities. We all can find ways to move more without doing anything we have to call "exercise." If you can move more in your daily life, you will always have a built-in way to exercise. For example, park at the far end of the parking lot and walk the distance. Take the stairs instead of the elevator. Get up to change the channels on the TV set. Get off the bus one or two stops early and walk the rest of the way. Get a dog. Having a dog is an automatic incentive to take several walks every day. An added plus: Studies show that having a pet is in and of itself good for your physical and mental health. So if you've always wanted a dog, now might be the time to get one.

Reward yourself. Consider keeping an activity journal. Each day record what you did and for how long. Buy some gold star stickers and give yourself one if you manage to exercise thirty minutes for five days in one week. Treat yourself to a movie, a magazine, a phone call to someone you love, or a nice bath. Do not make food a reward.

Take care of yourself. If your activity involves mostly walking, make sure your shoes are comfortable and supportive. If you need to buy new shoes, shop for them at the end of the day, when your feet tend to swell. Bring the socks you will normally wear with the shoes. Try on several pair and walk around in them. If possible, walk on a hard surface, not just on carpet. There should be about a thumb's width between the front of your toes and the front of the shoes. Your heels should not slip. The shoes you choose should feel comfortable immediately. Don't try to break them in—you could get blisters!

Monitor your blood sugar. Exercising is a powerful way to lower your blood sugar. When you exercise, check your sugar before and after to see how it responds. You may also need to check it more often over the next day. Since exercise can lower your blood sugar for up to 12 hours afterwards, your sugar the next day may be lower than usual. By checking your blood sugar after you exercise, you not only monitor for hypoglycemia (*see Chapter Seven*), but you also have a way of seeing how exercise is helping you.

Get a pedometer. This is a small device that counts each step you take. Pedometers cost about $14, and are becoming a popular way of encouraging physical activity. A reasonable goal is to take 10,000 steps a day. When you see how close you are to your goal, you will probably find creative ways to take more steps.

Ease yourself into it. If you really don't feel like exercising even though you know you should, try this little trick. Break your exercise down into tiny steps and do just one at a time. For example, suppose your exercise is walking, and you suddenly decided it's too cold and you'd rather pay bills, read catalogues, make phone calls, or do almost anything rather than take that darn walk. Just make yourself put on your walking shoes. That's it. No pressure. Just put on the shoes.

That was easy. Now maybe you could just step outside and see if it really is so cold.

Once you're outside, you might as well walk to the end of the block. Once you've walked the block, you might notice that it's not so bad. You might as well do the whole walk. You can reward yourself when you get in by calling a friend, drinking a cup of tea or reading a magazine.

Stick with it. Exercise has a way of becoming addictive. If you get yourself moving, especially if the activity fits into your routine and you like it, the positive effects of exercise will make you feel so good over time that you soon won't be able to do without it.

Precautions

Avoid injury. Start short and slow. It's better to start very slowly and work your way up than to start too quickly, do too much, and get injured. If you get hurt, you will have to recover—and this could set back your physical activity for who knows how long.

Use proper protective gear, such as a helmet when bicycling, goggles when playing racquetball.

Monitor your glucose if you are on medication. Exercising will probably lower your blood sugar. Be aware of this so you can check your finger sticks afterwards. You may need to lower your dose of insulin or medication, or you may need to eat a snack. If you find yourself eating more on a regular basis to ward off hypoglycemia, talk with your health care provider about adjusting your medication.

Protect your heart. Exercise is generally good for your heart. However, starting physical activity when you've been sedentary can strain your heart. Since people with diabetes have a higher risk of heart disease, the American Diabetes Association recommends an exercise stress test if you are over thirty-five years of age. Ask your doctor.

Protect your feet. Wear supportive athletic shoes for weight-bearing activities. Make sure they fit well. Examine your feet before and after exercise, and every evening at bedtime.

Protect your eyes. Diabetic retinopathy is a disease in which the blood vessels in your eyes are prone to leakage. This can ruin your eyesight. Activities that are rough and jarring, such as jogging, are not recommended if you have diabetic retinopathy.

Obstacles

People have many reasons for not exercising. Some of these are excuses; some are valid. Either way, your health depends on your ability to exercise, so let's figure out how to overcome some obstacles you might have.

Time. We live in a fast-paced society. Many of us have more roles and responsibilities than we can handle. If you are dealing with a new health problem like diabetes—getting used to the new regimen of blood tests, regular meals, shopping for and preparing food—finding more time to get out and exercise may seem like a joke. If this is the case, incorporate exercise into your current daily activities, and aim for a total of thirty minutes a day.

Dangerous Neighborhood. Unfortunately, many of us live in neighborhoods where we're afraid to linger outside. If walking in your neighborhood is going to make you the target of crime, that's not good for your health and we do not advise it. Perhaps you can walk somewhere else that's safe. Or ask someone to walk with you. Also, consider joining the local YMCA. And there's always the stairs; take any staircase you can. Walking up and down stairs is good aerobic exercise. Many people use this as their *only* aerobic activity and successfully lose weight and get in shape.

Weather. Rain, cold, or extreme heat are other reasons to stay indoors. Don't let these weather conditions keep you from being active. Have an alternate plan. If you can afford it, join an indoor gym. Some gyms, such as the YMCA, offer discounts for low-income individuals.

A free alternative is to find an indoor mall and briskly walk through it.

Consider exercising despite the weather. Don't do anything dangerous, but a little rain won't hurt you. Walk with a hood or an umbrella. Ideally, you'd swim to stay cool when it's hot, and jog to stay warm when it's cold.

"I'm too tired to exercise." As strange as it seems, the more active you are, the more energy you will have. As we mentioned earlier, exercise increases your levels of the mood-elevating hormones. Exercise helps lower your blood sugar, which, as long as it doesn't get too low, will help you feel better. Exercise increases your endurance and muscle strength. If you feel fatigued, ask your doctor to rule out medical causes. When you've been cleared, go ahead and exercise: Chances are you will have more energy than before.

"I'm too out of shape, or too old, or too sick." Even if you are confined to your bed, exercise is likely to benefit you; exercise will help keep your joints flexible and your muscles strong. Check with your doctor. There are exercises you can do even if you are confined to a bed or a wheelchair. These can help your balance, your strength, your flexibility, and your outlook. You can do leg-lifts

while in bed. You can lift small hand weights. If you have trouble walking, try swimming or water aerobics. Many gyms (such as the YMCA) and community pools offer water workout classes. Check with the ones in your area to find the best water workout for you. Remember, you can be fit and healthy whatever your age or size.

Getting off Track. Slipping up is normal. If you don't exercise for a while, don't beat yourself up about it. You can think about the problem and make some strategies; this way, if it happens again, you will have a plan to keep exercising. Think of a slip-up as a message that you need to fine-tune your routine.

EXERCISE RESOURCES

· Community pools

· Dances

· YMCAs

· Senior centers

· City programs and leagues

CHARLENE GETS MOVING

Charlene's doctor was strict about her need to exercise, so she reluctantly thought about it over the next week. She went out and bought some sneakers at the mall. On Monday, she decided to walk during her lunch hour, and have lunch afterwards at her desk. To her surprise, two co-workers asked if they could join her. Although they walked briskly up and down the five blocks near their office, they still had enough breath to talk. After a few weeks, Charlene realized she was really looking forward to these walks. She had made some new friends and her clothes were looser. Best of all, instead of needing to take additional medication, she was able to lower her dose!

Summary

- Regular exercise has many health benefits.

- Talk with your health care provider about the best exercise regimen for you.

- A good rule of thumb is to walk half an hour, five days a week.

- Monitor yourself and your blood sugars.

- Start slowly, increase gradually, and stick to it.

CHAPTER SEVEN

HYPOGLYCEMIA: THE MOST COMMON EMERGENCY SITUATION

BRIAN SAVES THE DAY

B*rian was on his way back from a business trip. The flight was overcrowded and stuffy, and delayed. They'd been on the runway for an hour. The crew had served beverages, but Brian knew they wouldn't serve food until they were in the air. Luckily, Brian was prepared and had brought a sandwich for a snack. He knew traveling made meals unpredictable and, now that he was on medication for his diabetes, he couldn't afford to have hypoglycemia. The man sitting next to him was complaining loudly about the delay. Brian couldn't help noticing that the man was on his second alcoholic drink. "It's going to be a long flight!" Brian thought. The man was shouting for the fight attendant, his voice slurred. He started demanding that the meal be served. He stood up and became more and more agitated. The attendant called the pilot and everyone began to stare. Brian wasn't sure if he should help restrain the man.*

But Brian glanced at him, and he noticed a red flash at his wrist. Brian recognized it as a medical alert bracelet. "He has diabetes!"

Brian shouted, immediately realizing what the man's behavior was all about. The man wasn't drunk; he was hypoglycemic. Brian urged him to take several of the candies he kept with him at all times. By the time the pilot got there, the man was calm and very embarrassed. The flight attendant quickly got him a tray of food.

HYPOGLYCEMIA

Hypoglycemia means your sugar has dropped too low and it is the most important diabetic emergency you should know about. In the story you just read, Brian kept the situation from getting dangerously out of control by recognizing the symptoms of hypoglycemia. The man, on the other hand, made a few mistakes. For example, he drank alcohol, instead of eating. However, he really did something smart, too: he wore a bracelet identifying himself as someone with diabetes.

Your health is your business, and you may not want to announce your health issues to the world. However, if you are unconscious for any reason, it is imperative that the people around you know that you have diabetes. If left untreated, hypoglycemia can eventually cause unconsciousness and seizures.

You should know how to recognize and treat hypoglycemia in its early stages. If you wait too long to treat hypoglycemia, your thinking can become affected. You won't know how to help yourself. Anyone on medication for diabetes could get hypoglycemia. Hypoglycemia is sometimes called an *"insulin reaction,"* but you can get it whether you are on insulin or on pills.

How low is too low? Hypoglycemia is technically defined as a blood glucose lower than 60. However, the blood glucose level at which *you* feel hypoglycemia may be slightly higher or lower.

We have spent most of this book discussing how to make

changes in your life in order to take care of your diabetes. Many of these changes mean that you need to have more structure in your life. You need to eat three meals a day, take your medication every day, check your blood sugar routinely, and see your health care provider regularly. But, even for the most careful people, life doesn't always cooperate. There will be times when the unexpected happens. In this case, it's best to have a back-up plan. Think of it as insurance. That way you have a plan B even if things do go wrong.

Hypoglycemia is a common result of unexpected little upsets in one's diabetic routine. You are at risk for hypoglycemia if you:

- Are late for a meal or miss a meal

- Eat less than usual

- Exercise more than usual

- Are under stress

- Increase your medication

- Are a women in certain phases of her menstrual cycle

You may also be at risk if you drink alcohol on an empty stomach, according to the American Diabetes Association. They recommend limiting yourself to one drink a day if you are a woman and two if you are a man.

If you have to make any changes in your eating/medication/exercise routine, the best way to avoid hypoglycemia is to check your blood sugar more frequently. Also, check your blood sugar as soon as you have any symptoms of hypoglycemia, which include both physical and mental signs. The symptoms usually start out as mild, gradually becoming more alarming.

Some physical symptoms of hypoglycemia are:

• Feeling shaky

• Breaking into a cold sweat

• A rapid heartbeat

• Feeling faint

• Feeling clumsy

• Sudden hunger

• Sudden fatigue

• Headache

Some mental symptoms of hypoglycemia are:

• Difficulty concentrating

• Dizziness

• Confusion

• Slurred speech

• Lack of coordination

• The feeling of being "out of your body"

• Emotional changes: sadness, anger, giggling

Once you have the mental symptoms of hypoglycemia, your judgment could be affected. This could be very dangerous. You should not drive or operate heavy and/or dangerous equipment if you have *any* symptom of hypoglycemia. Stop, take candy or glucose tablets, and don't continue until you feel back to normal. If in doubt, take a sugar tablet. If you let the hypoglycemia go untreated, you could lose consciousness and you won't be able to treat yourself. Consequently, your sugar will keep getting lower and your brain, which needs sugar to survive, will "starve"—leading to unconsciousness or death.

At this stage hypoglycemia can cause:

• Unconsciousness

• Seizures

• Death

BRIAN GETS STRESSED OUT

Brian's hard work was paying off. He was one of just a few people up for promotion. Although he was confident about his good work, he was still very nervous the day of the interview. He felt jittery and his stomach felt funny. He was in a rush and he didn't eat all his breakfast. As the hour of the interview grew closer, Brian felt kind of shaky and sweaty. He knew he was stressing over the interview, but he wondered if he could be hypoglycemic. Luckily he had time to check his blood sugar before the interview. It was 170. Brian was impressed that all those symptoms that sounded just like hypoglycemia were actually from stress. But he was kind of relieved that his sugar was fine. As soon as he got into the interview and started talking to his potential supervisor, he calmed down. And a few days later, Brian learned he had gotten the job!

Stress can feel like hypoglycemia. When you are under stress, your body releases *adrenaline,* your "fight or flight" hormone. This hormone makes your body feel jumpy, preparing you to take sudden action. Scientists believe it helped our ancestors escape dangerous animals in the savanna. In this case, when stressed, the released adrenaline works on your tissues to help release more glucose—which can be extremely useful. Glucose is useful. If you need to take some immediate physical action, you need some immediate fuel—glucose. Strangely enough, hypoglycemia also leads to production of adrenaline, so adrenaline makes your body feel the same whether the adrenaline is being stimulated by stress or by hypoglycemia. So if you are sweating and shaking and have a pounding heart beat, you might not know if it's from stress or hypoglycemia. Further, if you are under stress, you might not eat right. So, just in case, it's always a good idea to check your blood sugar.

If you are hungry or if your blood sugar is rapidly decreasing, you could also have symptoms like those of hypoglycemia. The only way to know is to check your blood glucose. If your glucose is in the normal range (over 60), but you just don't feel right, check again in 15 minutes. This way, you can make sure that your sugar isn't on the way down to hypoglycemic levels.

Don't delay treating your hypoglycemia. If you are experiencing symptoms, check your sugar as soon as possible before taking a sugar tablet to see if you are actually hypoglycemic. However, if it's not possible to check your sugar immediately, take some form of fast-acting sugar just in case. If you take a few extra sugar tablets it will raise your blood sugar, but not to a dangerous level. On the other hand, if you don't take the tablets when you need them, your sugar could continue to drop, and you could become confused and unconscious.

HYPOGLYCEMIA: EMERGENCY SITUATION STRATEGIES

Keep treatment for hypoglycemia handy at all times.

Luckily, you can treat most cases of hypoglycemia with something as handy as five to seven Lifesavers™ candies. Other recommended treatments are:

- Six jelly beans

- Ten gumdrops

- Two or three glucose tablets

- Four to six ounces of orange juice (a small glass or carton)

- Four to six ounces of soda (half a can); not diet soda!

- 1/4 cup raisins (one small box)

- Two lumps or two teaspoons of sugar

Always keep a source of fast-acting sugar in your car. Accidents are a serious and possibly fatal consequence of hypoglycemia. You never know when a traffic jam or a change in schedule can leave you trapped in your car. That is the wrong time to get hypoglycemic!

Any of the fast-acting forms of sugar should raise your blood glucose by about 25–50 mg/dl within fifteen minutes. If not, take a little more sugar. Don't treat hypoglycemia with sweets that have fat in them, such as chocolate, a milkshake, or ice cream. The fat in food slows digestion. In the case of hypoglycemia, you want to digest the sugar as quickly as possible! After taking your fast-acting sugar and checking your blood sugar fifteen minutes later, either eat a meal or have a snack within the next half hour.

If you are so severely hypoglycemic that you are drowsy or unconscious, other people should not force food or drink into your mouth. The food could go down into your lungs. Unless they can get you to take the food yourself or they can inject you with glucagon (sugar), they should call 911. Teach anyone living with you, even young children, to call 911 if they find you unresponsive. It could save your life some day.

Glucagon

If you live with someone else, you should keep a vial of glucagon (a prescription-only replica of the hormone that causes the liver to release stored sugar) in the refrigerator. A family member or roommate should learn how to give you glucagon in case you have severe hypoglycemia and lose consciousness. It could save your life. Injecting glucagon is not difficult. Once given, you should wake up within a few minutes. If not, the person who gave it to you should call 911.

If your mind is impaired by hypoglycemia, you are at a higher risk of having automobile and other accidents, as well as at higher risk of becoming angry and having poor judgment. Sometimes the change in your personality is something only a loved one may notice. (For example, he or she may notice that you get crabby.) On the other hand, you might feel rightfully annoyed about something and it's up to the other person to suggest that the problem might really be your low blood sugar. In fact, because your judgment can be so bad during a spell of hypoglycemia, it's in your best interest to teach the people around you what to do in an emergency. While you are under the spell of hypoglycemia, you might in fact refuse treatment. They are going to have to be tough and persistent to get you to check your sugar and/or take some glucose tablets.

We said that hypoglycemia might masquerade as crabbiness. It can also make you appear to be "drunk." As in Brian's story at the beginning of this chapter, hypoglycemia can make people angry and make their speech slurred and their actions clumsy. Sound familiar? If you don't know better, these could just be the behaviors of a drunk person. To make matters more complex, alcohol can worsen hypoglycemia. Alcohol keeps the liver from turning some of its stores into glucose. So someone could have alcohol on his breath, but his strange behavior could actually be due mainly to hypoglycemia.

Hypoglycemia Unawareness

Sometimes you can have hypoglycemia and have no warning signs. This is called *hypoglycemia unawareness*. Hypoglycemia unawareness doesn't usually happen until someone has had diabetes for fifteen-to-twenty years. As we learned in Chapter Twelve, diabetes can eventually affect nerves. Hypoglycemia unawareness is the result of decreased reactions by the autonomic nervous system—which controls that "fight or flight" response we talked about. If your autonomic nerves are not functioning normally, you may no longer feel the rapid heart rate or shakiness that hypoglycemia causes. The danger is that, without a warning sign to tell us to eat something sweet, our sugar can go lower and lower. People with hypoglycemia unawareness may not realize any problem until they are confused or become unconscious.

If you think you might be having periods of hypoglycemia unawareness, you need to discuss this with your health care provider. The best solution is to check your blood glucose levels more frequently—especially at times when your sugar is likely to dip. Fortunately, if people are able to avoid hypoglycemic episodes for several weeks, some ability to detect hypoglycemia can return.

Nighttime hypoglycemia

This is another instance in which you might be hypoglycemic and not know it. By nighttime hypoglycemia, we mean you have hypoglycemia while you are asleep. Nightmares can be a symptom of nighttime hypoglycemia. If you are suspicious that you might have nighttime hypoglycemia, you need to wake yourself up in the middle of the night and check your glucose. You should also check your glucose at bedtime. Call your health care provider to discuss adjusting your medication if you find you are experiencing nighttime hypoglycemia.

HYPEROSMOLAR SYNDROME

This emergency is much less common than hypoglycemia. In hyperosmolar syndrome, your sugar levels are extremely *high*— 600-1000 mg/dl or more! This situation occurs mainly if someone becomes ill and dehydrated. When your body is dehydrated, your sugar can go higher than normal, and it can cause you to become confused or unconscious. It is a very dangerous situation and is, at times, associated with death, but it comes on gradually. The people at most risk for hyperosmolar syndrome are the elderly sick who are not getting attention or who may be too weak to get enough fluid into their bodies. These people get progressively weaker, more confused, and eventually end up in a coma.

Other people at risk are those who have diabetes, but don't know it. If they get so sick that they are too weak to get fluids, they could develop hyperosmolar syndrome.

The treatment for hyperosmolar syndrome is intravenous fluids and hospitalization. Again, this is a very serious situation. If you get hyperosmolar syndrome, your body is often so stressed that you may die.

The best way to stay out of trouble is to keep checking your finger sticks if you are ill, to stay in touch with your health care provider, and to have family members or friends look in on you.

KETOACIDOSIS

Diabetic ketoacidosis is an emergency that is much more common for people with type 1 diabetes. It is caused by the production of acids when there is no insulin in the body. People with type 2 diabetes can develop ketoacidosis if they have severe infections or injuries that have put their body under extreme physical stress. Your sugar does not have to be particularly high to get ketoacidosis nor is it something you can detect using your glucose meter. Because of this acidic state in your body, ketoacidosis is very dangerous. It needs to be treated in an intensive care unit with insulin and fluids, under careful observation.

How do you avoid ketoacidosis? If you are sick, keep taking your medication and keep checking your glucose. If it is over 300, contact your health care provider.

Remember:

- Try to avoid situations that bring on hypoglycemia.

- Check you finger sticks regularly.

- Know the warning symptoms of hypoglycemia.

- Treat the symptoms as soon as possible.

- Wear a medical alert ID.

- Let people around you know you have diabetes and make sure they know what to do if you have a hypoglycemic attack.

CHAPTER EIGHT

TAKING CONTROL OF YOUR HEALTH

DARRELL CHECKS HIS SUGAR

Darrell ran his own construction company. It was stressful work. There was always some problem: materials didn't arrive on time, workers didn't show up, the client asked for last minute changes, and so on. Darrell took his diabetes in stride and took his medication regularly. That's why he was surprised when his doctor told him that his blood glucose was very high. Darrell had felt fine! The doctor increased his medication and pressured Darrell to start checking his own blood glucose. Darrell had learned how, so he made time for it every morning. He started seeing how his blood glucose changed. It seemed to depend on what he'd eaten the day before. Now he had a daily incentive to eat better. He decided he had time for that.

Diabetes is a disease that affects your whole body, so, naturally, when you have diabetes, you have to take good care of your body. Of course, people who don't have diabetes should also take care of their bodies, but they often don't. Too many people eat bad diets or smoke; they don't exercise, get medical checkups, see their dentist, floss their teeth, and have mammograms. Think of diabetes as an incentive to take really good care of yourself. The better you take care of your body, the better it will take care of you. Eventually, you could very well be in better health than the people who don't have diabetes!

In this chapter we'll discuss care that is specific to diabetes, and we will then review the key areas of your body that need attention. Of course, in addition to following these special care programs, you need to practice basic healthy habits like everybody else.

WHY IT'S IMPORTANT TO CHECK BLOOD SUGAR

Anyone on medication for diabetes should check his blood sugar (blood glucose levels) regularly. Even if you're not on medication, checking your blood sugar has several advantages. It:

- Allows better control of diabetes (studies have shown that people who check their blood sugar have better control).

- Gives you feedback so you can take the appropriate action.

- Keeps you out of danger.

- Lets you know how new foods affect your sugar.

- Lets you know how exercise affects your sugar.

- Helps you adjust your medication.

TAKING CONTROL OF YOUR HEALTH

With your blood glucose results, you and your health care provider can better adjust your medication.

In short, checking your blood sugar gives you more information, so that you can make informed decisions. For example, you will be able to tell exactly how that bag of popcorn has affected you.

Most importantly, checking your blood sugar gives you advanced warning if your sugar is going too high or too low. This way you can take quick action to prevent problems. For example, it's a good idea to check your blood sugar level before you go driving. Becoming hypoglycemic while driving can put you at risk of a car accident. Checking your blood sugar before you drive keeps you and your passengers safe.

Checking your sugar can also encourage you to keep exercising. If you see how your sugar drops after you exercise, this will motivate you to exercise more. If you see it dropping too low, you can take action fast and eat something.

What should my sugar levels be?
Check with your health care provider. For most people, the blood sugar should be:

- 80–120 before meals

- 100–140 before bedtime

Why is my sugar too high?
If your blood sugar is too high, these might be some of the reasons:

- **Food.** Eating too much or too soon before you check your sugar can cause a higher reading.

- **Hormonal**. Women can have higher sugar levels around the time of their menstrual cycle.

- **Stress**. If you're stressed out, it can raise your blood sugar.

- **Illness**. If you are sick, your numbers can rise.

- **Medication**. You might need a higher dose or you missed one.

Why is my sugar too low?

A low sugar is usually less than 60. This is called *hypoglycemia* and can make you feel terrible. It can also be dangerous. (For more about *hypoglycemia,* see Chapter Seven).

What should I do?

If your blood glucose is over 200 or under 60 on several occasions, call your health care provider. Otherwise, keep a record and discuss it with her at your next visit.

GLUCOSE METER

Glucose meters are the best way of getting an accurate idea of your blood sugar. When you use a meter, you prick your skin with a *lancet* to draw a tiny drop of blood. This is usually done from the fingertip, but it can also be done from other areas of the body, such as the forearm. You then place the drop of blood on a *test strip*, which is a small piece of paper that has been chemically treated to measure your sugar. You then insert the strip into the meter, which gives you a blood sugar read-out. Some newer devices automate this process for you.

You should record your blood sugar results along with the day and time. This is important information for you to share with your health care provider in deciding how well your diabetes is being managed. Some meters even have memories that will store your glucose results for you. There are many meters on the market, with a variety of options. Ask your health care provider for guidance in choosing the one the fits your needs.

When you are choosing a meter, consider:

- Ease of use

- Cost of supplies

- Special features, such as memory

- Insurance coverage

Manufacturers are constantly improving glucose meters. Many meters can now download your glucose results to a computer, and allow you to track your results over time. Someday soon, you may be able to skip the lancet all together. Companies are developing meters that can measure blood glucose through the skin. (However, at this point these meters are still not very accurate.)

Using the meter

Meters are very accurate if used properly. Ask your diabetes educator to review how to use your particular meter with you. Read the instructions. You will need to have the right technique and your meter needs to be calibrated. You will also need to keep the meter clean and make sure your test strips have not expired. With practice and the right technique, you can minimize the pain of pricking your finger and know your blood sugar results at any given time.

Caring for your body head to toe

When you have diabetes it's especially important to pay attention to your body. Concentrate on the following areas:

- Lifestyle

- Blood pressure

- Cholesterol

- Feet

- Eyes*

- Skin

- Teeth

- Stress

We'll go over them one-by-one now.

LIVING A HEALTHY LIFESTYLE

Checking your blood sugar regularly and paying attention to areas of your body that could become trouble spots are things diabetics have to do—and most diabetics get used to it. You can begin to be a good patient right now by vowing to respect your

---

* We will be going into more detail on the eye and eye complications with diabetes in Chapter Ten.

body. Eat food that is good *and* good for you. Keep your body strong and in shape with regular exercise. Don't drink to excess and do avoid drugs all together.

Don't smoke
Smoking causes heart disease, as well as lung cancer and emphysema. Smoking also damages the blood vessels to your feet. If you have diabetes and smoke, you're asking for trouble. In the past ten years, several treatments have become available that make it much easier to quit. If you have trouble quitting, speak to your doctor. We can now combine prescription and nonprescription medications to give you the best chance ever of kicking the habit. Talk to your doctor about what would be best for you. Whatever you do, don't put off quitting. This is one of the single most important steps you can take to live a longer and healthier life.

PROTECT YOUR HEART

Having diabetes increases your risk of getting heart disease. African Americans have the highest death rates from heart disease of any group in the United States. According to the American Diabetes Association, two out of three people with diabetes eventually die from heart disease or stroke. Minimize your risk of heart disease by keeping your diabetes under good control and by being alert for other risk factors. This means keeping tabs on your blood pressure and cholesterol and not smoking. Experts recommend that everyone with diabetes take a daily aspirin unless a medical condition prevents it. Check with your doctor.

High Blood Pressure

If you have diabetes, you probably have high blood pressure (hypertension) as well. Seventy-five percent of African Americans and 70 percent of White Americans with diabetes have high blood pressure. High blood pressure for diabetics and people with kidney disease is defined as a blood pressure 130/80 or greater. Because high blood pressure and diabetes each increase your risk of heart disease, doctors recommend that people with diabetes keep their blood pressure below 130/80.

> *If you have diabetes, you probably have high blood pressure (hypertension) as well.*

High blood pressure can also cause:

- Kidney damage

- Strokes

- Heart failure

If your blood pressure is too high, your health care provider will first recommend a healthier diet, exercise, and weight loss. If these steps don't lower your blood pressure enough, the next step is usually medication. Today, there are a vast number of blood pressure medications out there. Your doctor can pick one to maximize its benefits and minimize any side effects.

Diabetes with high cholesterol

Cholesterol is a type of fat normally present in your blood. Your health care provider should check your cholesterol along with some other types of fats. Together, these fats are called *lipids*. The main lipids are the *lipoproteins* (LDL and HDL) and *triglycerides.* As with high blood pressure, lipid problems increase your risk of heart disease and often accompany diabetes.

You have the best chance of avoiding heart disease if your:

- LDL cholesterol is less than 100.

- HDL cholesterol is more than 45 for men and more than 55 for women.

- Triglycerides are less than 150.

If your lipids are not what they should be, the initial treatment is diet, exercise, and weight loss. Again! If these don't sufficiently improve your lipid profile, you should allow your doctor to add the medication he thinks is best for you.

Diabetes with high blood pressure and high cholesterol

For many people with diabetes, it doesn't rain, it pours. These people not only have diabetes, but they also suffer from high blood pressure *and* unhealthy lipids. Any one of these conditions can raise an individual's risk of heart disease. When these conditions are grouped together, the risk increases significantly. Researchers are noticing that a growing number of people suffer from these combined conditions. These people also seem to be overweight, with most of their excess weight around their waists, so that they seem "apple-shaped" rather than "pear-shaped." Scientists have named this cluster of unhealthy conditions *metabolic syndrome.* It's important to recognize this syndrome and treat it aggressively. This is particularly the case for African Americans, since they are more likely to die from heart disease.

YOUR FEET

Compared to your heart, your feet don't seem that important—until you develop a foot problem and realize how much you depend on them. Having diabetes puts you at risk for amputations of your feet and legs. Most leg amputations begin with seemingly minor foot sores. The best way to prevent these consequences is to take excellent care of your feet.

Basically, diabetes affects the nerves and blood vessels in your feet, which results in problems with healing. This, in turn, can turn a minor problem into something big. For people with diabetes, an otherwise minor problem, such as a touch of athlete's foot, can lead to big-time trouble. Make it a daily habit to look at your feet, including the areas between all your toes. Be sure to dry your feet between the toes. Look for any redness and peeling skin. Redness can be a sign of infection; peeling skin can mean athlete's foot, a fungal infection that occurs more commonly in people with high blood sugar. If, for any reason, you are concerned call your health care provider for a check up. Do not treat foot problems yourself. This is really an area for which you want expert input.

Never walk barefoot. If you use public showers, say, at the gym, make sure you wear flip-flops. Shake out your shoes before putting them on at the beach, to dislodge any bits of sand; these can cause foot ulcers. Never use a heating pad. Never purchase shoes that are uncomfortable. And, even if you do purchase comfortable shoes, change them after about two hours to give your feet a rest.

If you do develop a foot ulcer or infection, don't despair. Medical science is developing new ways to help heal these problems, but do be prepared for the ulcer to take a long time to heal.

During this time, it's crucial to stay in close contact with a doctor or nurse who specializes in wound healing.

PROTECT YOUR SKIN

Keep your skin well moisturized—as long as you know that there is no infection present. Your skin acts as a barrier to protect you. Overly dry skin contains tiny cracks. Bacteria and funguses can enter these and cause infection. When you shower or bathe, don't use deodorant soaps; they are harsh and can dry out your skin. Use a moisturizing soap instead. Afterwards, apply moisturizer to your entire body while it is still damp. Pay particular attention to your feet. Call your doctor if you notice any problems.

SEE YOUR DENTIST

People with diabetes are more likely to get gum disease. This can cause pain, infections, and loss of teeth. Minimize your risk of gum disease by keeping your blood sugars under control, brushing twice a day, and flossing at least once a day. Regular teeth cleaning in your dentist's office also keeps your gums healthy. You should have your teeth cleaned at least twice a year.

GET A HANDLE ON STRESS

Stress can literally make you lose control of your blood glucose. When we are under stress our body produces hormones that help us react. As we discussed earlier, these have been called "fight or flight" hormones because they help us fight or run. But the same hormones can kick in during an unpleasant work interaction, even though we probably shouldn't fight or run—which increases our blood sugar. You may notice that during a period of stress, your sugars get out of control even when you are doing your part to take care of yourself. If this is the case, you may need to increase your medication under the guidance of your health care provider.

Of course, when we are often under extreme stress, we don't feel we have the time to take care of ourselves. So another reason stress could make your sugars worse is that you might let your diet slide, or you might feel too worn out to exercise. Try not to let this happen; it won't make you feel any better. If you do lose track of your healthy habits, come back to them as soon as possible.

Treat stress by scheduling relaxing activities. Take a walk, take a bath, garden, or listen to music. Do whatever works for you. You can also learn to meditate or do breathing exercises. Talk with your health care provider about other ways to beat stress.

Female Hormones

Women have another situation involving stress and hormones to consider. The hormonal changes that happen before your period can make you feel stressed out, causing you to eat poorly or not exercise. For some women, the hormonal changes of the menstrual cycle lead to temporary increases in their sugar. Keep track of your blood sugar and see if you notice a pattern.

Remember:

- Check you blood sugar regularly.

- A glucose meter gives you the most accurate reading.

- Pay attention to the key areas of your body: blood pressure, cholesterol, feet, eyes, skin and teeth.

- Try to live a healthy lifestyle and reduce stress.

CHAPTER NINE

WORKING WITH
HEALTHCARE PROVIDERS

ROBERT SEES A NEW DOCTOR

*R*obert had diabetes for a few years when he got a notice from his HMO that he had been assigned to a new doctor. He liked old Dr. Cooper and wished he'd had a chance to say goodbye. But Robert wanted to take care of his health, so he decided to go in for a checkup. The doctor breezed into the room, half-an-hour late. She shook Robert's hand and looked through his chart. She asked him about his medications, which he found annoying because they were listed in his chart. She seemed awfully young to be a doctor. Maybe she was one of those residents. She did a pretty thorough physical and gave him a lab slip. Robert found himself back in the waiting room, totally confused. He had forgotten to ask her about those strange feelings he was getting in his feet. He didn't know if or when he was supposed to come back, and he didn't know what the lab test was or when he should get it. He grumbled to his wife that he didn't care much for the new doctor. His wife asked the doctor's name, but Robert couldn't remember. He missed old Doc Cooper.

YOUR HEALTHCARE TEAM

Your team is made up of the medical professionals who care for you. They may or may not be a formal group. If they aren't, you yourself need to keep track of them. Either way, you are the "co-captain" of your healthcare team; your doctor is the other "co-captain." The following are the health care providers you might deal with when you have diabetes:

Primary care provider

Your primary care provider (PCP) will usually be a doctor, but may also be a nurse practitioner, or a physician assistant. The provider is a "generalist" responsible for taking care of most of the medical issues you will face. He or she will have experience in a wide range of medical problems, and also know when to refer you to a specialist, be it a physician or a diabetes educator.

Nurse Educator

The nurse educator will teach you the skills you need to manage your diabetes. She will often work overtime with you. For example, a nurse educator might work with you to fine-tune your medication.

Dietician

Your dietician will help you find the diet that is best for you. As we saw in Chapter Four, knowing what to eat when you have diabetes can get very complicated. Your dietician should be registered by the American Dietetic Association; he or she should be able to help you regulate your diet over time. You will need to be able to check with him or her periodically to monitor your progress and to answer your questions.

Ophthalmologist

An opthalmologist is a medical doctor who has done several years of specialty training in the diagnosis and treatment of eye problems. You should see one at least yearly for a special eye exam.

Podiatrist

A podiatrist spends years learning about the diagnosis and treatment of foot problems. He or she is licensed to perform foot surgery, if necessary. Your primary care provider may refer you to a podiatrist if you are having foot problems that require specialized attention, such as calluses or corns. Never treat these problems yourself!

Endocrinologist or Diabetologist

Endocrinologists specialize in hormonal diseases, including diabetes. Diabetologists specialize in diabetes. Most people with type 2 diabetes do not need to see either. Because diabetes is so common, health care providers are generally well trained in type 2 diabetes and can also help you with all your other health care needs. They can integrate your health care in a way that a specialist often cannot. Your health care provider may call the specialist for advice in your case or refer you to one. Consider seeing a specialist if your diabetes is not controlled by your primary care provider.

Diabetes support group

Your support group can give you valuable advice infused with personal experience. Your health care provider may suggest a group allied with his or her hospital; you may be a member of a church that sponsors a diabetes support group. You can also find a group by contacting the American Diabetes Association. If you have internet access, you are also certain to find online chat groups. Just be sure to check out any information with a reputable professional.

THE PATIENT'S JOB

As one of the team leaders, you are responsible for taking care of yourself. You need to take care of your body. You also need to do your part to make sure your interactions with the medical system go as smoothly as possible.

When dealing with your health care providers:

- Keep your medical appointments and be on time.

- Know your doctors' names.

- Know your medications and doses or keep a list in your wallet.

- Let your doctor know about other health care providers you have seen and any changes they have made in your treatment. Be sure he or she knows about any changes in your medications or in the dose of medications.

- If you don't feel right about a health care provider, get a different one.

- Wear an ID bracelet that identifies you as having diabetes.

TALKING TO DOCTORS

*Sadly but truly, at this time, many Americans, urban and rural, aren't
receiving the quality of medical care they need and deserve. Still, it's
useful for you to know how your relationship with your doctor might
work in a perfect world. By keeping that ideal alive, we can perhaps
bring it closer. What follows, then, is an account of an ideal situation
that is now available to only about one-third of the nation.*

You should be able to trust that your health care providers know
what they are doing and that they want to help you. Doctors are
actually "only human;" they have good days and bad days. Some
are old and some are young. Some are outgoing and some are
more reserved. Some run like clockwork, some always run late
(sometimes that means they'll spend more time with you; sometimes that means they are too busy). But whatever their habits,
they should always be courteous.

Your relationship with your doctor is very important. You
need to be able to tell him or her personal information. You need
to be able to trust your doctor with your life. Give it a few meet-
ings, but if you don't feel right about your doctor, consider
switching. Having said that, let's bring in reality: Health care
providers will not know everything. But they should be able to
look it up or ask if they don't know something. In this world of
quickly changing information, you may even learn a few things
yourself, on the internet, on TV or in the newspaper before your
health care provider does.

Let's also be realistic about time. You should not feel rushed;
you should get all your questions answered. On the other hand,
your health care provider generally has just so much time for your
appointment (usually fifteen to thirty minutes). During this time

the two of you should catch up on any new issues. Go over lab tests, do any relevant physical checks and review medications. It's a lot to get done. To ensure that the appointment goes as well as it can, do your part. This includes being on time, having a written list of things you would like to discuss, and knowing if you need to ask for a refill of your medication. You also need to know your medications and doses, and your finger stick glucose values. If your glucose meter has a memory, bring it along so your health care provider can review the numbers.

Sometimes there is just too much to discuss in one appointment. This is not just a matter of time. Even if you had unlimited time, its hard to learn too many new things at once. If you have unfinished business, make sure you and your health care provider can agree on when you will talk again, either by phone or at the next visit.

You should feel comfortable asking any question to your health care provider. Don't protect his or her feelings. You should also bring up anything that you are unhappy about. Often the health care provider can correct the problem or at least explain the "whys." You also need to be truthful about your own behavior. If you are having trouble staying on the diet, you should admit it. If you forget your medication doses, tell the truth. Otherwise, your health care provider might increase your medication, or prescribe a different one—when all you really need is a system to remind you to take it. Remember, it's your body and your health. You are the leader of the health care team. The other members are there to help you.

At the end of every visit you should know:

• How your diabetes is doing.

• What dose of medication you should be on.

It's a good idea to take some notes so you can remember what the plan is. You might also want to bring a companion to help you think of questions while you are in the doctor's office. Often, you will hear so much information that it helps to have someone else to remember facts and ask questions.

- When you are next to go to the lab—and what you'll be getting tested for.

- When your next doctor's appointment will be.

- What the follow-up is for any other problems you might have. (For example, if you have a sore on your foot, you should know whether the podiatrist will contact you or whether you are expected to phone the podiatrist.)

It's a good idea to take some notes so you can remember what the plan is. You might also want to bring a companion to help you think of questions while you are in the doctor's office. Often, you will hear so much information that it helps to have someone else there to remember facts and ask questions.

FIRST MEETING WITH A MEMBER OF YOUR TEAM

Chances are that you will need to get to know more than one person in your health care team. Perhaps you will have a physician and a nurse educator *and* a dietician. It can be overwhelming getting to know all these different people and figuring out what their role is in your health care. Here are some tips to keep things straight. Remember, as the co-leader of your health care team, these are things you have a right to know and need to know.

- Ask for their business cards. If they don't have one, write down their name, phone number, and what their job is. You also have a right to know if the doctor is only there temporarily or if the doctor is in training.

- Keep your health care provider's name and phone number next to your telephone at home, and keep another copy in your wallet.

- Ask how they will help you and under what circumstances you should make an appointment or call.

- Find out how to best reach them.

- If it is practical for you, ask if you can communicate with them via e-mail or in writing.

ROBERT TAKES CHARGE

Robert asked the receptionist for his new doctor's name. It was Dr. Clark. He decided to give her another chance. At his next visit, he was on time and prepared. Dr. Clark was on time, too. This time, when she went over his medications, Robert knew them. He realized that Dr. Clark was just making sure that he was taking what she thought he was taking. Then, when she asked him if there was anything he wanted to discuss, he pulled out a list he had made up. He wanted to know if his sugars were good enough. He mentioned the tingling in his feet. He wanted to know about getting a flu shot. He wanted to know about a diet he had heard of. And he wanted to know about an herb his cousin was taking.

Dr. Clark told him she wanted to concentrate on his feet and his sugars. She said she'd have to look up the herb and the diet and get back to him. She also told him that the flu shots weren't available yet, but that it was *time for his yearly eye exam. Robert guessed that would be okay. He asked her if she would answer in writing, by phone, or let him know at the next visit. They agreed that she'd phone him by the end of the week. Dr. Clark examined his feet carefully and told him that, although they looked fine, the tingling might be caused by a neuropahy (nerve damage). His sugars were also higher than they should be. They agreed that he'd increase his medication and call Dr. Clark with his finger stick results in one week.*

Robert checked his list: 1.) His sugars were too high; he'd increase his medication and call the nurse with his finger stick results. 2.) He had the number of his eye doctor and would call him for an appointment. 3.) Dr. Clark would call him next week with the answers to his other questions. 4.) He would see Dr. Clark in a month, but he'd call her sooner if the tingling in his feet got any worse.

Robert left the office feeling much better about his new doctor.

STAYING ON TOP OF THINGS

After you have gotten to know everyone and have been through the initial teaching sessions, and if your sugars are well-controlled, your care will settle down into a routine. Your team will probably ask you to do periodic tests depending on your circumstances. The American Diabetes Association recommends the following care schedule:

At Each Visit:

- **Weight**. Your weight directly affects your blood sugar control. You should be weighed at each office visit.

- **Blood pressure**. Because 70 percent of people with diabetes have high blood pressure, and because diabetes and high blood pressure are a double risk for heart disease and kidney failure, high blood pressure needs to be caught and treated early. Your blood pressure should be checked at every office visit. Ask your health care provider what your blood pressure should be. For most diabetics, it should be less than 130/80.

- **Foot exam**. Taking good care of your feet is crucial. Diabetes can cause problems with the nerves and blood vessels in your feet. It can also lead to poor healing. As a result, people with diabetes are at risk of not noticing small injuries, such as blisters, on their feet—that can quickly turn into dangerous infections. For this reason, you need to carefully wash and dry your feet and inspect them daily. You should never walk barefoot. Your health care provider should look at your feet at each visit.

Every Three to Six Months:

- Have a scheduled visit with your primary care provider.

- Have your HbA1c tested. HbA1c stands for hemoglobin A1c, or "glycosylated hemoglobin," which measures glucose that sticks to your red blood cells. Since the lifespan of a red blood cell is three months, this is a good measure of your average glucose during this time. This measurement is different than that of your blood glucose. For example, a normal fasting blood glucose is less than 100. A target HbA1c for diabetics is 6.5 or less. You should have your HbA1c checked every three months.

A DIFFERENT TEST

Fructosamine is a blood test that can check for your average blood glucose over a period of about two weeks. Your health care provider may choose this test instead of the HbA1c when adjusting your medication.

Every Year:

- **Kidneys.** Diabetes can harm your kidneys, leading to kidney failure and the need for dialysis. To catch any problems, the American Diabetic Association recommends a yearly microalbumin, a urine test to see if the kidneys are leaking small amounts of protein, an early sign of kidney injury.

- **Lipid panel.** High cholesterol combined with diabetes puts you at very high risk for a heart attack. So it's a good idea to periodically check your cholesterol. A lipid panel checks your cholesterol and the levels of "good" cholesterol (HDL) and "bad" cholesterol (LDL).

- **Eye exam.** Diabetes can lead to problems with your eyesight, including blindness. You should see an ophthalmologist every year. The eye doctor will use drops to enlarge your pupils to look inside your eyes to check for any complications that might be caused by diabetes. He or she will also check for glaucoma.

  See your eye doctor sooner if you notice any problems with your eyes or vision.

- **Flu shot.** Usually available starting each October, the flu shot can either prevent the flu or make it milder if you get it. People with diabetes can get sicker with the flu. And since the flu can lead to fatal pneumonia, it's a good idea to get your flu shot every year.

Every One-Two Years:

- **For women**: Have a gynecological check up and talk to your doctor about birth control. If there is any chance you will become pregnant, the more planning you can do with your physician is better for your baby. During pregnancy, the baby's development is extremely sensitive to your glucose levels, so many women go on insulin for the duration. Pregnant or not, all women need periodic gynecological check ups.

Ask Your Doctor About:

- **A heart checkup**. The American Diabetes Association recommends an exercise stress test for people over thirty-five with diabetes who plan to start exercising.

- **The pneumovax shot**. You should get this shot to ward off the bacteria that causes the most common form of pneumonia. This pneumonia is still often fatal. The pneumovax can also prevent some types of meningitis as well as sinus infections.

This is a basic list. If you are at risk for other problems or if there is a concern about a specific problem, you might have different tests or more frequent tests. And, if you are having any new symptom or problem, you may have different or more frequent tests as well.

IF YOU ARE ADMITTED TO THE HOSPITAL

It's more difficult to stay in control if you are hospitalized. Because hospital personnel work in shifts, you may interact with a different doctor every day, and you could be assigned a different nurse every eight hours. This can be confusing. Remember, there is still *one* doctor who is primarily responsible for your care. Make sure you know who that is.

Remember:

- You have a healthcare team. You're the co-captain and your doctor is the other co-captain.

- Taking care of your diabetes means checking your glucose regularly.

- Check your diabetes "target body zones" daily.

- See your health care provider regularly and follow the recommended testing schedule.

- Learn how to communicate effectively with your health care providers.

CHAPTER TEN

MEDICATIONS FOR DIABETES

REGINA TAKES ACTION

Regina was worried about her blood glucose levels. She walked her dog every morning and went to an aerobics class twice a week. She had really improved her diet, and she had lost twelve pounds over the past six months. Still, her fasting blood glucoses were over 170. She was disappointed that she wouldn't be able to control her sugar without medication, but her main goal was to get her sugars down. She made an appointment with her doctor to get some medication.

If you have diabetes and need medication, you may feel unfortunate. But there is a bright side. Never before have we had so many different ways to treat diabetes, and known so much about how to minimize long-term complications.

Improvements in diabetes care have arrived at an accelerating rate. If you had diabetes in the early 1900s there wasn't much that you could do. Insulin wasn't available until 1921. But when it arrived, it changed everything. The discovery of insulin was a remarkable achievement, saving millions of lives. Indeed, development of insulin as an injected medicine won its creators the Nobel Prize. It took over thirty years more before the first pill to treat diabetes was invented in 1955. By the late 1980s and 1990s, there were a rush of new medications, all of them attacking diabetes in a variety of ways. Depending on your particular situation, you can now find the medication that is best for you.

Before we discuss to the various pills available for diabetes, let's talk about taking medication in general. Medication is only effective if taken in the prescribed way. For the best success, follow these rules:

- Continue a healthy lifestyle.

- Communicate with your doctor.

- Know your medications' names.

- Fine-tune your regimen.

Let's go over these one-by-one:

Continue a healthy lifestyle
Taking medication instead of optimizing your diet and exercise won't work. If you slack off on your diet and exercise regimen, you are likely to have uncontrolled blood sugars and gain weight.

Communicate with your doctor
If you are given a new medication, make sure you understand whether you are supposed to continue the old one, stop it, or decrease the dose. Write down the instructions or ask for them in writing.

Bring your pill bottles to appointments. If your doctor has changed your medication dose, have him ask the pharmacy to change the instructions on the label to avoid confusion.

Before you begin any medication, tell your doctor about all of the other medications you are taking. This includes diet supplements, over-the-counter medications, and vitamins. Each can have serious interactions with your medication. If you are seeing more than one doctor, make sure that each one knows your "medication resume."

Know your Medications' Names
Medications almost always have two names: the generic name, which is based on the chemical composition of the drug (and may be hard to pronounce), and the brand name, which is usually shorter and catchier. You should learn both names for any medication you take; one medication can go by several different brand names. Health care providers might use either the brand name or the generic, and you need to recognize what they are talking about.

- Memorize your medications and doses.

- Take your medications on schedule.

- Keep your medications organized in a pillbox.

- Keep a record of your medications in your wallet. This will help doctors and paramedics in case of an emergency. It can also help jog your memory if you forget.

- Read the package inserts that come with your medicine. They generally list every possible thing that could go wrong. Be aware of the possible problems, although some of the problems they list are very rare. Ask your health care provider or pharmacist about common or serious side effects.

Side Effect or Allergy?

Some side effects happen when you first start a medication, but soon resolve or clear up. Some continue, but are tolerable. Some are a sign of a problem. If you notice any new symptoms after you begin a medication, check with your health care provider.

A side effect is different than an allergy. Typical signs of an allergy are a rash, itching, or difficulty breathing. If you experience any of these, stop the medication and call your doctor immediately. The difference between side effect and allergy is important because, if your reaction is an allergy, it can become worse if you are exposed to the same medication again.

A word of caution: once you take a medication, whether a pill or insulin shots, you are at risk for hypoglycemia. Hypoglycemia is also known as an "**insulin reaction**" but you don't have to be on insulin to suffer from hypoglycemia. Hypoglycemia means your blood sugar has gone too low—lower than normal and lower than is necessary for your body and brain to function. (*See Chapter Seven.*)

Fine-tuning your regimen

- Take your pills even if you feel well.

- Take your pills even if you *don't* feel well, but call your doctor and check your sugar.

- Don't take someone else's medications. Your friend may tell you about a wonderful new medicine she's taking and urge you to try it. Or you may have seen a convincing ad on TV. But everyone is different. You run the risk of serious side effects if you don't check with your doctor first.

Some fine-tuning questions:

When do you need to change medication? There is no "best" pill or treatment for type 2 diabetes. The best pill for you will depend on your own personal health characteristics. You may need to try more than one type of pill, a combination of pills, or pills plus insulin.

Even if diabetes pills do bring your blood glucose levels near the normal range, you may still need to take insulin if you have a severe infection or need surgery. Blood glucose levels tend to increase during times of physical stress, and pills may not be able to adequately control your diabetes.

If you plan to become pregnant, you will need to control your diabetes with diet and exercise or with insulin. It is not safe for pregnant women to take any of the diabetes pills.

Are you on too much medication? If you are taking many pills and you need them all, you are not on too much medication. However, sometimes your doctor can reduce the number of pills you're taking by prescribing pills that are more effective.

You are on too much medication if it is causing your sugar to go too low much of the time.

THE PILLS

Doctors call the pills used to treat diabetes *oral hypoglycemics.* "Oral" means by mouth. "Hypoglycemic" refers to a low blood sugar. Thus, oral hypoglycemics are medications you can take by mouth to lower your blood sugar.

Oral hypoglycemics are not insulin and they can't take the place of insulin. They only work if the pancreas is still making some insulin. Some hypoglycemics stimulate the pancreas to produce more insulin; others make cells more sensitive to insulin. Some prevent the elevation of sugar.

For this reason, none of the oral hypoglycemics are of any use for people with type 1 diabetes, whose pancreas doesn't make insulin. However, for many people with type 2 diabetes, the pancreas, while working, is still not capable of producing enough insulin for the body's needs. In these situations, oral hypoglycemics are less effective and insulin may be necessary. People with type 2 diabetes are most likely to benefit from oral hypoglycemics if they are of normal weight and have not had diabetes for more than ten years.

Why not take an insulin pill? Because insulin is simply not available in pill form. If taken by mouth, insulin is destroyed in the stomach by our digestive enzymes. However, research is under way to create forms of insulin that don't require injection.

Oral Hypoglycemic Medications

Sulfonylureas

The first diabetes pills to be invented were the *sulfonylureas,* introduced in 1955. A military physician discovered them by accident. He had noticed that soldiers who were given certain sulfur-containing antibiotics developed low blood sugars. He used this side effect to help people with diabetes—and the sulfonylurea medications were born.

The sulfonylureas are the oldest pills for diabetes and probably still the most widely prescribed. They work by stimulating the pancreas to release more insulin. The pancreas has to be able to produce some insulin for sulfonylureas to work, so they are ineffective in type 1 diabetes. In most cases, they work well for type 2 diabetes but, eventually, they seem to lose their effect. This is because the pancreas slows down its insulin production.

The sulfonylureas have been divided into two *generations*. The second generation is newer, more powerful, and more expensive.

Sulfonylurea side effects:
All sulfonylureas can cause hypoglycemia (*see Chapter Seven.*) This is more of a problem with longer-acting versions and with the stronger second-generation pills. Sulfonylureas often cause weight gain.

Sulfonylurea Medications:

First Generation:	Generic Name	Brand Name
	tolbutamide	Orinase®
	tolazamide	Tolinase®
	chlorpropamide	Diabinase®

Second Generation:	Generic Name	Brand Name
	glyburide	Micronase®
	glipizide	Glucotrol®
		Glucotrol XL®
	glimepiride	Amaryl®

Metformin

Metformin, the only biguanide in common use, goes by the brand name Glucophage®. It's been in use around the world for over twenty-five years, but it was not approved in the United States until 1995. Metformin stops the liver from making too much glucose and it may increase the sensitivity of muscle cells to insulin. Because metformin does not increase insulin levels, it does not cause hypoglycemia if used by itself.

Metformin is often used in combination with sulfonylureas or with insulin.

The most *serious* side effect of metformin is a condition called *lactic acidosis,* a fatal reaction that seems to only occur in people with certain conditions, such as kidney problems, liver disease, congestive heart failure, or severe peripheral vascular disease. Your doctor should make sure you don't have any of these conditions before prescribing metformin.

The most *common* side effect of metformin is gastrointestinal upset. Stomach upset, diarrhea, and abdominal pain can occur in up to 30 percent of patients. These stomach problems are less severe if metformin is started at a low dose and increased gradually.

Metformin also has some beneficial side effects. Unlike the sulfonylureas and insulin, both which cause weight gain, metformin can cause weight loss. This side effect is very helpful for the many overweight people with type 2 diabetes. It is also beneficial on cholesterol profiles.

Thiazolidinediones (also known as the glitazones)

These include rosiglitazone (brand name: Avandia®) and pioglitazone (brand name: Actos®). They are increasingly being used, and are now recommended as the first-line treatment of type 2 diabetes. They are the first medications to directly reverse insulin-resistance, the basic problem in type 2 diabetes. Thiazolidinediones do this by increasing cell sensitivity to insulin; they work their changes slowly and the full effect can take up to three months. Because thiazolidinediones are slow-acting, if you were on another oral hypoglycemic drug when you started taking thiazolidinediones, you will probably be advised to initially continue both medications.

A side effect of the thiazolidinediones is that they can cause potential liver problems. Because of the potential for liver inflammation, periodic blood tests are recommended. Some people also have troublesome leg swelling. The drugs may also cause mild anemia. Rosiglitazone may decrease the effectiveness of birth control pills.

The thiazolidinediones *don't* cause hypoglycemia if used alone.

Another potentially beneficial side effect is that thiazolidinediones can improve fertility. This is because insulin resistance decreases fertility; the thiazolidinediones reverse that effect.

Glucosidase inhibitors (acarbose)

Acarbose goes by the brand name Precose®. Acarbose slows the digestion of carbohydrates. Normally, enzymes must break carbohydrates down into simple sugars to be absorbed through your intestines because they cannot absorb them. If acarbose is taken with a meal, carbohydrates are converted into sugar more gradually. The sugar then passes into your bloodstream more slowly, and your blood sugar rises less abruptly. But acarbose does not lower blood sugars as well as many other oral hypoglycemic medications.

Acarbose, too, has side effects. The sugars are eventually absorbed lower down in your intestine, causing gas, abdominal pain, and diarrhea in 75 percent of people taking the medication.

This problem is alleviated if acarbose is begun at a low dose and slowly increased.

The Meglitinides

This group of medications goes by the names repaglinide (brand name: Prandin®) and nateglinide (brand name: Starlix®).

Like the sulfonylureas, the nateglinides cause the pancreas to release more insulin. Their advantage is that they are shorter acting and can be taken right before a meal.

Like the sulfonylureas, the meglitinides can cause hypoglycemia.

Remember:

- A variety of oral medications can treat type 2 diabetes.

- Review with your doctor how to take the pills properly.

- Review the ways to detect and treat hypoglycemia. (See Chapter Eleven for more detail)

- Wear an ID tag that identifies you as having diabetes.

- Despite the variety of pills for type 2 diabetes, many people will eventually need insulin.

ALL ABOUT INSULIN

GREG STRIKES A BARGAIN

*G*reg wasn't feeling too good. He'd been up half the night urinating, a routine that had been going on for a week. He felt tired and cranky. He'd controlled his diabetes just fine with diet, exercise, and medication for years. But now his blood glucose was measuring over 250. At his appointment with his nurse practitioner, she told him that his HbA1c was too high. After reviewing his diet and exercise, she suggested he add some insulin to his medications. Greg was skeptical. He'd been fine on the pills. He hated the idea of shots. He promised to exercise more and to return in two weeks.

INSULIN

In 1921, doctors gave the extract of a ground up cow pancreas to a little girl who had been dying of type 1 diabetes. The girl made a miraculous recovery and insulin treatment was born.

Since that time, insulin has been refined so that we have different forms with different actions. But despite the millions of lives insulin saved, today we don't often think of it as the wonderful innovation it was. Now that there are a variety of diabetes medications that people can take by mouth, many people hate the thought of taking insulin. They worry that it is painful. They see it as a sign that their diabetes is worse.

Needing insulin does not mean that you have developed type 1 diabetes. The usual reason that a person with type 2 diabetes begins taking insulin is that their pancreas cannot make enough insulin for their insulin-resistant tissues. Despite the maximum doses of oral medication taken, their sugars are still too high. Eventually, about 40 percent of people with type 2 diabetes end up on insulin. They still have type 2 diabetes and are making some insulin of their own. It's just not enough. Why does this happen? It's probably a combination of the tissues becoming more insulin-resistant and the pancreas slowing down its insulin production.

The good news is that, once you're on insulin, you may be surprised at how well you feel. Another surprise: The needles don't really hurt much at all. They are so tiny that thinking about getting a shot probably hurts more than the shot itself!

GETTING STARTED

When you start taking insulin injections, there's a lot to learn. Be sure that you have a good teacher, someone you can call if you have any questions. Many health care facilities employ a special diabetes educator who can teach you all about administering your insulin—how to store it, how to give yourself a shot, and how much to use.

Types of Insulin

When you get your insulin, you should keep two key pieces of information in mind: *the time of action* and *the concentration.*

Time of Action

This has three key periods:

- Onset: How long the insulin takes to begin its effect.

- Peak time: When the insulin has its greatest effect.

- Duration: How long the insulin keeps working.

Be sure you know the onset, peak time, and duration for the insulin you are taking. This is how you know when to take the insulin in relation to your meals.

Normally our pancreas secretes insulin throughout the day. The amount of insulin is finely-tuned according to what we eat. No insulin regimen is as good as what our body could do if we didn't have diabetes. *However, the goal of insulin treatment is to approximate how our pancreas works as much as possible.* To that end, scientists have developed different formulations of insulin that kick in at different times after an injection.

The main types of insulin in order, from shortest to longest-acting:

Lispro This is the shortest-acting insulin. Lispro was introduced in 1996. It is absorbed quickly and acts quickly. So that you won't have to plan ahead, you can inject Lispro right before you eat. Because of its short duration, it has less risk of resulting in hypo-glycemia.

Regular This was the first formulation of insulin available. Until 1996, it was the only short-acting insulin available. Its onset of action is 45 minutes. You need to take Regular 30–45 minutes before meals.

NPH and Lente These are insulins that have been bound to a protein to slow down their absorption. Their onset of action is intermediate. The extra protein makes them cloudy in appearance. To be absorbed properly, you need to remix the bottle by rolling it gently between your hands.

Ultralente Ultralente is long-acting. Its effects last up to 30 hours.

Glargine (brand name: Lantus®). Glargine lasts 24 hours with no peak time.

Premixed If you are on a stable regimen that doesn't change, you can get a pre-mixed insulin formulation. For example, "70/30" combines NPH and Regular insulin in a ratio of 70 units NPH to 30 units of Regular. This is especially helpful for people with poor eyesight.

Concentration

Insulin is commonly measured in units. The concentration of insulin we use in the United States is U-100. This means that in every milliliter of fluid, there are 100 units of insulin.

Other countries may use U-40 and U-500. (U-40 is less concentrated, with only 40 units of insulin in a milliliter; U-500 is more concentrated, with 500 units of insulin in a milliliter.) If

TIME OF ACTION OF THE VARIOUS INSULIN TYPES

Type	Onset	Peak	Duration
Lispro	Within 15 minutes	30–90 minutes	3 hours
Regular	30–60 minutes	2–3 hours	4–8 hours
NPH	1–3 hours	8–12 hours	14–24 hours
Ultralente	2–4 hours	Minimal	26–30 hours
Glargine	1–2 hours	Minimal	18–24 hours
70/30	30 minutes	2–12 hours	18–24 hours

you travel abroad, you can avoid confusion by bringing your own insulin. If you do end up having to get a different concentration, be sure to get the syringes made specifically for that concentration. For example, if you are given U-40 insulin, you should get syringes calibrated for U-40 insulin. This will help you avoid making the dangerous mistake of giving yourself the wrong amount of insulin.

Sources of Insulin

Nowadays, most insulin is "human" insulin, identical to the insulin we make ourselves. Past sources of insulin were the pancreases of pork or beef—which worked equally well. However, since some people have allergies to animal source insulin, the fact that scientists have used special genetic techniques to create bacteria that can produce human insulin has been an important advance.

Side Effects of Insulin:

- *Hypoglycemia.* Be careful when starting on insulin. Stick to your regular schedule of meals and exercise. Review the symptoms of hypoglycemia discussed in Chapter Seven. The treatment is the same as it would be for hypoglycemia related to pills.

- *Weight gain.* Insulin helps store glucose as fat. If your diabetes was out of control before going on insulin, you were losing some glucose in your urine. Now it will be used in muscle and the excess will be stored as fat. You may want to review your diet and exercise plan with your health care provider or dietician to be sure you're not consuming too many calories. If you are also on pills for diabetes, *metformin* can help minimize weight gain caused by insulin.

- *Increased appetite.* Some people notice a greater appetite when on insulin.

- *Allergy.* Insulin allergy is fairly rare. If you experience itching and redness at the site of injection, you might have an allergy to insulin—check with your doctor.

Giving yourself the shot

For many people, sticking themselves with a needle is the scariest part of going on insulin. The new insulin needles are lubricated, extremely thin, and very short. They are almost painless. Your health care provider or diabetes educator can review injection technique with you. With practice, giving yourself insulin will become as routine as flossing your teeth.

Injection technique:

- Swab the bottle and skin with alcohol.

- Draw as much air into the syringe as the amount of insulin you'll be taking.

- Roll the insulin bottle to disperse insulin evenly.

- Turn the bottle upside down.

- Plunge the needle into the bottle, pushing air into the bottle.

- Allow pressure to push the insulin into the syringe to the appropriate calibration (measurement).

- Remove the syringe from the bottle.

- Push the syringe plunger a little to force air out of the needle: you should see a drop of insulin at its tip.

- If the insulin has been refrigerated, warm it while in the syringe to room temperature to minimize pain.

- Inject quickly.

Rotating injection sites

To allow tissues to recover and prevent problems at the injection site, you should vary the area where you inject your insulin. Changing the site is referred to as "*rotating injection sites.*" Your injection sites should be areas of your body where there is a lot of fat under the skin. These areas include the abdomen, the thighs, the buttocks, and the upper arms. Try to stay within the same area at the same time of each day. Change the site from shot to shot. In other words, you might inject your abdomen before breakfast, but you would then inject a different part of your stomach each day.

Insulin is absorbed most quickly from the abdomen, less quickly from the arms, and slowest from the thighs and buttocks. Absorption from the abdomen is the most consistent.

Consistency means that your sugar will regularly drop at about the same time each day, allowing you to schedule your injections in relation to your meals. If you change sites, the time it takes your insulin to drop will change unpredictably.

Exercise will create more rapid absorption. For example, if you go running after injecting yourself in your thigh, your blood glucose might drop sooner than usual.

If necessary, you can give yourself an insulin shot through your clothing.

Use the appropriate syringe for the amount of insulin you are taking. In other words, use a smaller syringe if you are not taking as much insulin as usual so that the calibrations are more accurate.

Insulin pens are a convenient way to carry insulin. They come with insulin cartridges that you put into the pen. You then "dial" the amount of insulin you need. These pens are good for those people who might have trouble measuring insulin into a syringe.

If you can't deal with needles, there are a variety of other devices that might help—but they are expensive. Jet injection devices, for example, force insulin under the skin using a powerful blast of air. Insulin pumps utilize a needle that has been surgically put into your abdomen. Their benefit is that they can deliver continuous insulin. Because their bodies make their own insulin, type 2 diabetics wouldn't need to use an insulin pump.

Storing your Insulin

You don't need to keep your insulin in a refrigerator. In fact, room temperature is best if the vial will be finished within a month. If the room temperature is comfortable for you, your insulin will be fine.

Be sure not to shake, freeze, or overheat insulin. Doing so can break down its protein structure and make it inactive. Don't use insulin that has changed appearance—going from clear to cloudy—or if it has developed clumps. This may be an indication that your insulin has gone bad. You should also suspect that your insulin might be outdated if you find that it isn't lowering your blood glucose anymore.

GREG GIVES INSULIN A SHOT

The week after he saw his nurse practitioner, Greg had dinner with his brother-in-law, John. He remembered that John had been on insulin for his type 2 diabetes for a few years. John told Greg that taking the insulin had been tricky at first, but that he never felt better. John was very happy he had made the change. The minor inconvenience was more than made up for by how good he felt. He had more energy. His sugars were great. He had even traveled with insulin. The conversation made a big impression on Greg. He called his nurse practitioner a few days later and told her he'd decided to give insulin a shot.

Summary

- Many people with type 2 diabetes use insulin to bring their blood sugars to a healthy level.

- Insulin injections don't hurt that much.

- Learn the "onset of action" and the concentration of the insulin you are taking.

- Know how to recognize and treat hypoglycemia (*see Chapter Seven for more details.*)

CHAPTER TWELVE

LONG-TERM COMPLICATIONS OF DIABETES

D iabetes is the seventh leading cause of death in the United States. It's the leading cause of blindness, and the leading cause of kidney failure. People with diabetes are more likely to have heart attacks, strokes, and poor circulation; 60–70 percent of people with diabetes have nerve damage.

The statistics are frightening, but they are a warning, and not necessarily what will happen. Most of the complications of diabetes can be delayed or avoided altogether through good blood glucose control.

Diabetes care has improved greatly in the past several decades, but there are still too many diabetics whose blood glucose, cholesterol, and blood pressure are not as well controlled as they should be. The statistics *can* be improved.

The complications of diabetes increase the longer you have the condition and the higher your blood glucose has been. Most complications can be minimized by:

- Keeping your blood glucose, blood pressure, and lipids (fats) under control.

- Not smoking.

- Getting regular checkups.

Many of the complications we'll discuss in this chapter happen slowly and silently. In other words, you might feel great—while slowly going blind. Don't wait till you have a symptom. It could be too late by then.

The most common serious complications of diabetes are usually:

- Vascular disease (problems with the cardiovascular system).

- Retinopathy (problems with your eyes).

- Kidney failure.

- Neuropathy (problems with the nervous system).

- Infections.

RISKS TO YOUR CARDIOVASCULAR SYSTEM

Your cardiovascular system consists of your heart and all your blood vessels. Cardiovascular complications of diabetes include high blood pressure, poor circulation, strokes, and heart disease. This usually occurs from the hardening of the arteries, a complex reaction involving lipids, damage to the blood vessels, and inflammation, which doctors call *atherosclerosis.*

Hypertension, the medical term for high blood pressure, is extremely common in people with type 2 diabetes. Seventy-five percent of African Americans with diabetes have hypertension. Hypertension can be severe without causing any symptoms, so people don't know they have it unless they get their blood pressure checked. It is a major cause of health problems in the African-American community. It contributes to kidney failure, strokes, and heart failure.

Heart attacks occur because of blockages in the blood vessels that feed the heart oxygen and nutrients. Blockage of one of these can cause symptoms of chest pain or chest heaviness. Other symptoms are dizziness, rapid or skipping heartbeats, feeling sick to your stomach, or numbness of the arm. African Americans have a high death rate from heart attacks, so it's crucial to recognize these symptoms and to immediately call 911 if any occur.

Heart failure means that the heart is no longer able to pump blood as well as it should. The result is that fluid backs up in the lungs, while the brain and muscles are starved for oxygen. Symptoms of heart failure include dizziness, trouble breathing, fatigue, swelling of the legs, and loss of consciousness.

Strokes are due to blockages or bleeding in the vessels in the brain. You may have a warning sign of a stroke, such as numbness or weakness in an arm, a leg, or in your face. Other signs are dizziness and loss of consciousness. Strokes are medical emergencies. Their damage can be reduced with prompt treatment. If you experience any of the warning signs, you should call 911.

Poor circulation can cause pain in your feet and legs after walking. It can lead to poor wound healing and put you at risk for amputations.

REDUCING THE RISK

- Keep your blood sugar under control.

- Treat high blood pressure.

- Treat high cholesterol.

- Don't smoke.

- Get regular exercise.

Also, if you have atherosclerosis, your doctor may want to start you on aspirin treatment. Aspirin helps prevent hardening of the arteries by thinning the blood and reducing inflammation.

Your Eyes

Diabetes can harm your eyes in a variety of ways. Diabetes-related complications are the leading cause of blindness in the United States.

Retinopathy means damage to your retina. Your retina is the innermost layer of your eye, the area where a myriad of blood vessels and nerves converge. Only *ophthalmologists,* doctors with special training in diseases of the eye, have the skill, experience, and tools to reliably examine your retina. Retinal damage happens gradually, and you can already have irreversible damage without noticing any problems. Even if you don't have diabetes, it's a good idea to see an ophthalmologist at least once a year. If you have retinopathy, your ophthalmologist may recommend laser surgery. This can prevent your loss of vision from being as severe as it might otherwise be.

Glaucoma is the result of high pressure in the eye which can damage the optic nerve and lead to blindness. Glaucoma is more common in African Americans and also more common in diabetics. Glaucoma needs to be treated with special prescription eye drops before damage to the optic nerve occurs. Again, irreversible damage can occur before any warning symptoms.

Cataracts are another problem that diabetics especially have to watch out for. Cataracts are the result of cellular deposits forming within the lens of your eye. Your lens is transparent, but the deposits are not; consequently they block your vision. Cataract surgery removes the lens and replaces it with an artificial one. The surgery is simple and effective at restoring eyesight.

The treatment for cataracts is not urgent. In fact, doctors usually wait until cataracts are bad enough to affect vision before they remove them.

To save your eyesight, be compulsive about checkups. Because retinopathy and glaucoma can cause irreversible damage before you notice any symptoms, you should have an eye exam by an ophthalmologist when your diabetes is first diagnosed. You can then go once a year, unless your doctor advises more frequent checkups.

Again, keeping your blood glucose and blood pressure under control, as well as not smoking, will help minimize your chances of developing eye complications.

Your Kidneys

African Americans are more than twice as likely to get kidney failure. The reasons for this are unclear, but one reason is probably that African Americans have more high blood pressure than the general public. Having hypertension in addition to diabetes is an added risk for kidney failure.

Your kidneys filter your blood through tiny capillaries. All the blood in your body is continuously filtered through your kidneys to draw out waste products, which are then excreted in your urine. Your kidneys also regulate your water balance.

If your kidneys fail, you are unable to excrete waste products or fluid. These build up in your system. They can make you very ill, and even kill you. These problems can be treated by dialysis, in which a machine acts as your kidneys. However, a machine cannot adjust your fluid and chemical balance with the precision that your body can. Furthermore, dialysis requires you to be attached to a machine for several hours each week. Five percent of people with type 2 diabetes end up on dialysis.

A kidney transplant allows you to live a more normal life. But there is a waiting list for kidneys. Not everyone who wants or needs one will be able to get one. If you do get a transplanted kidney, you will need to take special medication to keep you from rejecting the transplanted kidney. Unfortunately, this medication may put you at risk for life-threatening infections and cancer. It can also make glucose control more difficult.

Minimizing your Risk of Kidney Failure:

- Keep your blood glucose close to normal. Studies have shown that this will help prevent kidney failure.

- Control your blood pressure. Eat a diet low in salt. If you need medication, take it faithfully.

- Don't smoke.

- Control your cholesterol.

- Have tests done regularly to check your kidneys' health. If your doctor suspects that there is a problem, she will perform a *microalbumin test* to check your urine for small amounts of protein. Normally, your kidneys don't pass protein. If there is more than a certain amount of protein in your urine this means that your kidneys are not well. A normal urine test can only detect a fairly large amount of protein. The microalbumin test specifically checks for tiny amounts of protein that are a signal of early kidney damage. If you treat this problem promptly, there is a chance of reversing the damage.

If your doctor detects protein in your urine, she will recommend you begin special medication that may stop or even reverse your kidney damage. Two groups of blood pressure medication have been helpful: the *ACE inhibitors* and the *angiotensin II receptor blockers.*

Neuropathy

Neuropathy means disease of the nerves. Sixty percent of people with diabetes have some problem with their nervous system. Risk factors for neuropathy are high blood glucose, age, alcohol excess, and height.

Our nervous system is a vast network of nerves with our brain as the command center. You can think of it as your body's electrical system. Nerves control the movement of our muscles. They provide *sensory feedback,* telling us:

- *Position:* that the ground beneath our feet is flat or steep.

- *Temperature:* that the bath water is too hot.

- *Fine touch:* that the object we feel in our pocket is a key rather than a coin.

- *Pain:* that we have just stepped on a thumbtack.

Our nervous system is continuously detecting and responding to vast amounts of information, usually on a subconscious level. It allows us to listen to music, to see a flower, and to walk.

We are even less aware of a specialized part of the nervous system called the *autonomic nervous system*. The autonomic nervous system runs a myriad of our bodily functions mainly without our awareness or control. It helps us breathe, assists our sexual functioning, helps us digest our food, help us expel our urine, keeps our heart beating, regulates our blood pressure, and controls when we sweat. Amongst its many responsibilities are our heartbeat, our breathing, and the contractions of our intestines.

Diabetes can harm any nerve in the body, but it most commonly causes damage to this autonomic nervous system (*autonomic neuropathy*) and to the peripheral nervous system, which is the area farthest from the brain (*peripheral neuropathy*).

One of the earliest symptoms of peripheral neuropathy is unusual sensations or lack of sensation in the feet.

It is important that your doctor test your nerve function in your feet. You could have significant neuropathy and feel fine, but having peripheral neuropathy puts you at risk for *amputations*.

Common consequences of peripheral neuropathy are:

- Foot pain or burning

- Foot numbness

- Difficulty in keeping your balance

Improve peripheral neuropathy by getting your blood glucose under good control. Reduce the risk of foot complications by examining your feet every day, never walking barefoot, and only buying shoes that fit well.

Autonomic neuropathy increases with time or poor glucose control.

Some complaints that might signal autonomic neuropathy are:

- Digestion problems, including bloating or regurgitation after eating. This occurs because the nerves controlling stomach emptying malfunction.

- Sexual problems. Men may have trouble with erections. Women may notice a loss of lubrication.

- Inappropriate sweating.

- Feeling dizzy whenever you stand up. This is because the nerves that tell your blood vessels to tighten to keep blood from rushing to your feet don't work.

Symptoms of neuropathy can often be improved by better blood sugar control. Otherwise the treatment depends on the problem.

The treatment for autonomic neuropathy depends on the organ involved.

The pain of peripheral neuropathy can be relieved to some extent by medications, both in pill and cream form.

Infections

A high blood sugar weakens your immune system. People with diabetes are more likely to get infections and the infections are more difficult to heal. Common sites of infection are the mouth, skin, lungs, ears, feet, and genital areas. Infections from any of these areas can spread. As with other long-term complications, avoid infections by keeping your blood glucose under control. Examine your feet daily and get regular medical and dental checkups. See your doctor at the first sign of any problems and get these recommended vaccines:

- A *pneumonia vaccine* protects you from the bacteria causing the most common type of pneumonia. This pneumonia kills thousands of people every year.

- A *flu shot* protects you from influenza viruses. It is prepared every year for the flu season, and is generally available in October. Flu viruses are apt to change, so you can still get the flu even if you've been vaccinated—but it should be milder. The flu can lead to fatal pneumonia, and kills many people yearly.

Summary

- Diabetes can cause many serious complications, but you can reduce your risk.

- Keep your blood glucose under good control.

- Don't smoke.

- Control your blood pressure.

- Get regular checkups.

- Pay attention to any new symptoms you may have.

CHAPTER THIRTEEN

DIABETES IN PREGNANCY

TASHA WANTS A BABY

Tasha had always wanted lots of children, but when she was diagnosed with diabetes she assumed she couldn't have any. She had once seen a movie in which the beautiful young star had diabetes. The star got pregnant against her doctor's orders, and she got sick and died. Tasha's husband just wanted what was best for her. The couple discussed their concerns with Tasha's doctor. He assured them both that it was safe for Tasha to have a baby, but that she would have to go on insulin. In fact, she would have to go on insulin **before** she got pregnant. And she might have to check her blood sugars up to eight times a day!

Tasha and her husband had very mixed emotions. They were excited at the prospect that they could actually start a family. On the other hand, they weren't sure they could handle the complicated schedule of insulin shots and checking blood sugars. Tasha worried that if she made a mistake her baby would be born with problems. She told Dr. Smith they'd have to think about it.

PLANNING A PREGNANCY WHEN
YOU HAVE DIABETES

With our current medical advances, women with diabetes have healthy pregnancies and deliver healthy babies all the time. But it takes some planning and lots of discipline. Women with diabetes do have an increased risk of delivering large babies. This might require the mother to have a Caesarean section and for the baby to be monitored in the intensive care unit after birth. However, if you are able to do what it takes to control your diabetes, you decrease your chance of complications. And, in case you were worried, your baby will not be born with diabetes just because you have diabetes.

But when you have diabetes, you *must* plan your pregnancy ahead of time. You should discuss your plans with your doctor and ask for her guidance. Your glucose control must be excellent before you conceive. Poorly controlled diabetes increases your risk of miscarriage and birth defects.

It really isn't okay to wait until you find out you are pregnant to control your sugar. The baby's internal organs form in the first four to eight weeks, before you even know you're pregnant. It's impossible to know you're pregnant for at least two to four weeks after conception, and often women don't know until longer than that. Meanwhile, the baby is forming and growing every day. By the time you find out you are pregnant, your baby could have suffered irreversible damage. This is why all experts stress that women with diabetes plan their pregnancies with care and have excellent sugar control *before* they become pregnant. After all, isn't the goal a healthy baby? Once you find out you are pregnant, you need to keep up the good work and continue controlling your sugar.

If you don't watch your sugar, your baby could be born:

• With serious lung problems

• With birth defects

• Mentally disabled

And you could develop serious problems with your:

• Kidneys

• Eyes

• Nerves

To this end, stay on birth control until you have controlled your sugars for several months and your doctor gives you the go-ahead to get pregnant. Review the checklist on the next page to see if you're ready.

YOUR PRENATAL CHECKUP

During your pre-pregnancy checkup, your healthcare provider will check for diabetes-related complications. Even women who already have diabetes-related complications can safely have babies, but they need to get the diabetes and the complications under good control first. Pregnancy can make your complications worse. The changes that take place in your body during pregnancy put a huge stress on your system. Your heart has to work harder to pump blood through you and the baby. Your kidneys have to work harder. You might develop high blood pressure. If you have retinopathy, it can worsen. With good care before and during your pregnancy, you minimize your risk of getting serious health problems. Amazingly, most of the physical changes go

PRE-PREGNANCY CHECKLIST

- Your doctor gives you the go-ahead

- Your health is stabilized

- Your sugars are controlled

- You have access to prenatal care with a high-risk pregnancy doctor, specialized in the care of diabetes

- You are on insulin if necessary

- You have a glucose meter and you know how to use it

- You can afford all the supplies for nine months

- You are prepared to check your blood glucose several times a day for nine months

- You are taking folic acid

- You don't smoke, drink or use drugs

- You have family and friends to help you out during the pregnancy and with the newborn

back to normal shortly after delivery. And your risk of developing complications after your baby is born does not rise if you have controlled your blood sugar during your pregnancy.

Your health care provider may put you on insulin, because all the pills available to treat diabetes can cause birth defects. Women who have been on pills will need to change to insulin before getting pregnant and for the duration of the pregnancy.

Even if you were able to control your diabetes without medication before you became pregnant, you may now have to go on insulin to get your glucose under the best possible control.

You will need to check your glucose several times a day. Your blood glucose goals are:

- Before meals   70–100

- Two hours after a meal   less than 140

Before you get pregnant, your health care provider will probably recommend that you begin taking folic acid, a vitamin that helps your baby's nervous system develop properly. As with glucose control, it's important that you begin taking folic acid before pregnancy because the baby's nervous system starts developing in the weeks before you even know you are pregnant.

Now is also a good time to quit smoking, even if you couldn't do it before. You should stop drinking alcohol. Review all your medications, including vitamins and herbs, with your health care provider to see if they are safe in pregnancy.

WHAT TO DO DURING YOUR PREGNANCY

· Keep your prenatal appointments.

· Check your blood glucose as directed.

· Gain the right amount of weight.

· Eat a healthy diet.

· Continue exercising.

FROM THE BEGINNING

Be prepared for hard work and discipline. Keep your eyes on the prize: a happy, healthy baby. All pregnancies can have morning sickness, fatigue, weight gain, strange rashes, etc. Added to that you may have to deal with forty weeks of checking your glucose several times a day. You may have to inject yourself with insulin two to four times a day. You will have to check in with your health care provider every two weeks.

Many experts recommend you check your glucose before and after meals, at bedtime and at 3 a.m. That nighttime check may be annoying, but remember, after your baby is born, you will be waking up at night more than once.

During pregnancy your sugars should remain:

- Before meals: 60–105

- After meals: less than 140

- Nighttime: 60–100

If your sugars are higher than 180 or even higher than 140 during several checks, call your health care provider. Your baby is changing and growing every day. Even a brief period of poorly controlled glucose could affect your baby.

If you are not able to control your glucose at home, your doctor may decide to hospitalize you for a brief period to control your glucose. Before you go home, you may get more intensive instruction and have a review of your diet.

You should meet with a dietician early in your pregnancy to help you choose nutritious foods and to guide you on how to gain the right amount of weight. Experts usually recommend a weight gain of 22–32 lbs. This extra weight supports the baby's growth.

If you are overweight, the recommended weight gain is less. It may be just 15 pounds. Remember, whether or not you are overweight, this is the wrong time to lose weight. You need some extra weight to help nourish your baby.

During your first three months of pregnancy, morning sickness can make it hard to stick to your diet. Morning sickness is worse when your stomach is empty, which is why it's common in the morning. (Some women feel morning sickness all day.) Obviously this can interfere with your meal schedule, and increase your risk of hypoglycemia. Try eating smaller and more frequent meals. Drink water between meals. Keep crackers at your bedside to take first thing in the morning.

Because your glucose needs are more intense, you will have an increased chance of becoming hypoglycemic. Check your glucose throughout the day and always check your glucose before you drive. Hypoglycemia has not been shown to hurt the baby. Apparently even if the mother's sugars are low, the baby is able to extract enough sugar from the mother's bloodstream. However, hypoglycemia can be harmful to you, and you need to be well to care for and protect your baby.

As you progress in your pregnancy, your weight increases and the hormones your body makes to support the baby increase. As this happens, you will require increasingly higher amounts of insulin. In fact, you may well be on more insulin than you've ever experienced. This doesn't mean that you will be taking more injections; it just means that you might need to inject a higher dose of insulin each time.

Because of the more intense insulin regimen, your health care provider might suggest you go on an insulin pump. These devices are a good idea for people who need to be on intensive insulin treatment. They are as safe and as effective as shots, and many patients feel they are more convenient.

During pregnancy, you should continue your folic acid supplement; your health care provider will also recommend calcium and iron supplements. Stick to the dose and preparation she recommends. Many commercial vitamin preparations have huge doses of various vitamins. This is not the time to take too much; it could harm your baby.

Unless your doctor tells you otherwise, continue exercising. Exercise is good for you and helps keep your glucose levels stable. It also keeps you in shape for delivery and for dealing with a newborn. However, don't start any new rigorous activity. Also avoid exercises in which you could fall or get hit, such as, jogging or racquetball. Check your sugar before you exercise, and keep some form of fast-acting sugar on hand in case of a hypoglycemia emergency.

THE EFFECTS OF HIGH BLOOD SUGAR ON YOUR BABY

Good blood glucose control decreases the risk of birth defects. Good glucose control also decreases the risk of the baby growing too large.

A big baby sounds like a healthy baby, but in this case that's not so. A baby exposed to too high a blood sugar from the mother can be big, but have poorly developed internal organs. Or a baby could have breathing problems. A large baby also makes delivery more difficult—which could result in brain damage.

During your prenatal visits, your obstetrician will check your baby's growth and progress with an ultrasound machine. If the baby looks like it's going to be too large, your doctor will recommend a C-section (a common recommendation for women with diabetes.)

If a baby has been exposed to high blood sugars, his own insulin will be working overtime and he is at risk for hypoglycemia after delivery. We discussed in Chapter Eleven the dangers of hypoglycemia to an adult. Imagine how hard it would be on a baby! These babies would initially need to be treated in the intensive care unit.

AFTER THE BIRTH

Congratulations, you have a new baby! Immediately after delivery, your body will begin the process of returning to its pre-pregnancy state. Your body is reversing the changes it went through over nine months, but it takes several weeks. Don't expect to feel quite like yourself during this time.

Be extra careful in checking your blood sugars. The rapid fall in hormone levels can make your blood sugars unpredictable. Breast-feeding can also lower your blood sugars, as can forgetting to eat because you are so busy with your new child. Keep snacks with you and stay in close touch with your health care provider. Remember your baby needs a healthy mom!

If you have decided to breastfeed, you will need to stay on insulin instead of your diabetes pills. Otherwise, you can resume caring for your diabetes as you did before you planned the pregnancy.

A word of caution: Don't have sex again until you get birth control. You can get pregnant at any time, even if you're breast-feeding.

DEALING WITH DIABETES AND A BABY

After you give birth, you need to take care of your diabetes and your body, which is recovering from your pregnancy and the birth of your new baby. Let other people help you with as many other tasks as possible: changing diapers, making meals, cleaning your house. Ask for, and accept help. You need to rest and recover and get to know your child!

As we already said, you can breastfeed if you have diabetes. In fact, breast milk is the ideal food for your baby and is cheaper and more convenient. You don't need to buy, mix and warm up formula, or wash bottles and nipples. Breastfeeding can also help lower your blood sugar and make it easier to lose weight. However, your sugars may swing more if you breastfeed. Check your blood glucose and have some fast-acting sugar handy while breastfeeding. Don't put the baby's feedings ahead of yours. You need to be healthy so that you can care for your newborn. When your baby feeds, have a snack, too.

Get back to your exercise regimen as soon as your doctor gives you the okay.

How is your mood? Even in the best of circumstances, lots of new mothers suffer from feeling sad after childbirth. This could be a form of depression called the *baby blues,* which is related to your hormones dropping. But if you have diabetes, it could also be hypoglycemia. Check your blood glucose to be sure you're not hypoglycemic. If you have blues that you can't shake, don't hesitate to talk to your health care provider.

GESTATIONAL DIABETES

Gestational diabetes means that, although you didn't have diabetes before, you develop it during a pregnancy. Gestational diabetes is the most common complication of pregnancy. Up to one in ten African-American women get gestational diabetes. They are twice as prone to it as White women. Being over twenty-five when you get pregnant, being overweight, and having a family history of diabetes also increases your risk.

RISK FACTORS FOR GESTATIONAL DIABETES

- Being African American, Latino, Native American, or Asian-American

- Being over 25-years-old

- Having a family history of type 2 diabetes

- Being obese (Body fat greater than 27)

- Having a previous miscarriage

- Having a previous baby over 10 pounds

All women should be checked for gestational diabetes as a routine part of prenatal care. This is usually done at the twenty-fourth to twenty-eighth week of pregnancy because gestational diabetes usually occurs during the second half of pregnancy, at about the fifth month. Your health care provider will do a special test called a glucose tolerance test. For this test, you will be given a special drink that is very sweet. An hour later your blood will be tested for glucose. If the level is 140 mg/dl or more, you might have gestational diabetes.

In gestational diabetes, your sugars are normal in the early part of pregnancy, so your child is at no increased risk of birth defects. However, if your sugars are too high in the second half of pregnancy, your baby is at risk for being too large, and may suffer problems during the birth and after.

Just like women who have had diabetes before their pregnancy, you need to take tight control of your sugars to give your baby the best chance in life. If your sugar is over 140 mg/dl, this means going on insulin for the duration of the pregnancy.

Huge hormonal changes occur in pregnancy, helping the baby grow inside you. The increased hormones in your system can cause insulin-resistance. In this way, gestational diabetes is similar to type 2 diabetes. After delivery, three out of four women have their sugars return to normal. However, of these, *half* will get diabetes later in life. All women who have had gestational diabetes should be checked for diabetes yearly.

What You Need to Know about Diabetes and Pregnancy

- With some planning, you and your baby have little risk of long-term problems.

- You must check with your doctor ahead of time if you have diabetes and want to get pregnant.

- Your sugars must be under excellent control *before* you get pregnant to prevent birth defects.

- You may need to go on insulin.

- You must get regular prenatal care.

- Gestational diabetes means diabetes that occurs because of pregnancy, but that resolves itself after the baby is born. It's twice as common in African-American women.

CHAPTER FOURTEEN

HOPE FOR THE FUTURE

GREGORY DOES HIS HOMEWORK

Greg was fourteen and had had diabetes for two years. He knew his classmates were curious about how he tested his sugars. At first, they had teased him, but not any more. When his biology teacher assigned the class to give presentations, Greg decided to talk about all the interesting advances in diabetes.

A diagnosis of diabetes is no longer a sentence to a life of disease and complications.

If you have diabetes, you now have access to an explosion of advances in treatment. People with diabetes have many more choices of medication than they ever had before. Insulin treatment has become increasingly sophisticated, more closely mimicking our natural insulin response.

Monitoring diabetes is more precise, and research is ongoing to make it less painful.

Here are just a sampling of the myriad technological advances currently underway:

FEWER SHOTS

Oral insulin: As it stands now, if you swallowed insulin, the acid in your stomach would break it down so that it became inactive. But scientists are experimenting with ways to protect insulin from being digested in the stomach. They are formulating a specially coated insulin pill that would pass through the stomach undigested. The coating would come off in the small intestine, where the insulin could be absorbed.

Inhaled insulin: Researchers are close to perfecting a form of insulin that can be inhaled. Like an inhaler for asthma, it would deliver insulin to the lungs where it would be absorbed. Another device might deliver an insulin mist that would be absorbed through the mouth.

An insulin patch: Scientists are developing patches that would use electrical currents, ultrasound waves, or chemicals to help transport insulin through the skin.

MORE MONITOR CHOICES

Painless meters: The ability of many new glucose meters to take blood from "alternative sites" decreases the pain of pricking your finger. The fingertips are more sensitive to pain than the arm, thigh, and abdomen. These meters also require less blood.

The GlucoWatch: This monitor senses your blood glucose using an electric current to pull blood through your skin. Although it is already on the market, it is not yet reliable enough to use without another meter. And it's expensive. At this point the GlucoWatch and supplies cost almost $6,000 per year.

Surgery

Pancreas transplantation: This has already been going on for decades. A pancreas from a donor who didn't have diabetes can produce insulin normally, effectively curing type 1 diabetes. However, there are drawbacks. As with any organ transplant, medication is required to suppress your immune system. These *immunosuppressive drugs* put you at risk for infections and cancers. For that reason, pancreas transplants are mainly done on people who also need kidney transplants and would be on the immunosuppressive medications anyway. Another problem is that there are not enough donors for pancreas transplants to meet the demand. Finally, while pancreas transplants can, in some cases, cure type 1 diabetes, it is not a solution for the majority of people with diabetes—those with type 2. Thus, although pancreas transplantation provides a more reliable insulin supply, it is not enough; we also need to improve insulin-sensitivity.

Treatments on the Near Horizon

Islet cell transplantation: Islet cells are the cells that make insulin. Islet cell transplantation involves infusing these cells into the body through an IV; they then proceed to make insulin in the recipient. Although recipients of these cells would still have to take immunosuppressive drugs, getting the cells through an IV is a minor procedure compared to the major surgery required to transplant a pancreas. Supply and demand is still a problem at this point, but genetic engineering might be able to create more islet cells.

Incretin peptides and dipeptidyl peptidase-IV: As we write, researchers are studying this new class of drugs for the treatment of type 2 diabetes. Incretin peptides and dipeptidyl peptidase-IV promise an injectable medication that will help control blood sugar and also have a beneficial effect on weight. They have not yet been approved, but are on the way.

Although research into the many genes responsible for type 2 diabetes is underway, it doesn't point to a cure. The best cure for type 2 diabetes is through lifestyle change, which is also an effective means of prevention. A case in point: The people who participated in the Diabetes Prevention Program were able to turn around their risk of diabetes.

The striking results from this program, as well, led to public health efforts to identify the millions of people with undiagnosed diabetes and pre-diabetes and to teach them the best way to keep diabetes at bay: by focusing on weight loss, a healthier diet, and physical activity.

So, while science and business combine to improve technologies for treating diabetes, while millions of dollars are spent, and while more research will help countless lives, the really hard work, the really necessary work, will be in something much more "low-tech." It will be in reversing our bad habits—in exercising, losing weight, and eating better. Reversing a bad habit is more difficult than popping a new pill, but it will benefit us more. As with most things in life, the best treatment is prevention.

This is not the first lifestyle-related epidemic Americans have dealt with. By educating people of the dangers of cigarettes, we have managed to decrease cigarette smoking. This was not done by any advance in technology, but by a good old change in habit. (The motivation to change this destructive habit came not just from willpower, but from changes in laws and public health policy. For example, laws prevent cigarette advertisements from appearing on television.)

Diabetes has become a great enough concern to the health of our communities that we should consider similar approaches. We can work to limit ads selling junk food to children. We can require our schools to emphasize healthy food in their cafeterias and vending machines. And we can adequately fund school physical education.

Remember, you do have control over your diabetes. By taking control of your emotions, your diet, and your activity level, by checking your sugars, keeping your medical appointments, and taking your medication properly, you can lead a normal, happy and long life. Best of luck to you!

DELICIOUS AND HEALTHY RECIPES FOR DIABETICS

All the recipes in this appendix are from the American Diabetes Association

Copyright © American Diabetes Association

Recipes excerpted from the following cookbooks: *Diabetic Cooking For Seniors, Flavorful Seasons Cookbook* by Robyn Webb, *Forbidden Foods Diabetic Cooking, The Healthy HomeStyle Cookbook,* and *The New Family Cookbook For People With Diabetes.*

Reprinted with Permission from *The American Diabetes Association.*

To order any of the books, please call 1–800–232–6733 or order online at http://store.diabetes.org.

BAKED CATFISH

An old Southern favorite, this breaded catfish is baked, not fried, to save calories and fat.

Number of Servings: 4

Serving Size: 4 oz

INGREDIENTS

Name	*Measure/Weight*
catfish, or ocean perch fillets (1 pound total), thawed if frozen	4 ea
white bread, crumbled, or 1 cup fresh bread crumbs	2 slices
grated Romano or parmesan cheese	2 Tbsp
chopped fresh basil or oregano	2 tsp
salt	1/2 tsp
pepper, ground black	1/4 tsp
egg beaten, or 1/4 cup egg substitute	1 ea
low-fat (1%) buttermilk	1/4 cup

PREPARATION INSTRUCTIONS

1. Preheat the oven to 400 degrees F. Prepare a baking pan with nonstick cooking spray.
2. In a pie pan or shallow dish, mix the bread crumbs, cheese, basil or oregano, salt, and pepper. Set aside.
3. In another pie pan or dish, combine the egg and buttermilk.
4. Dip each fish fillet first in the milk mixture, then in the crumb mixture, to coat both sides with crumbs.
5. Arrange the fillets in one layer in the baking pan. Bake 15 to 20 minutes, until the fish flakes easily with a fork.

Exchanges Per Serving	Nutrition Information Amount per serving	
1/2 Starch 3 Lean Meat 1/2 Monounsaturated Fat	Calories 225 Calories From Fat 98 Total Fat 11 g Saturated Fat 3 g Cholestrol 121 mg	Sodium 518 mg Total Carbohydrate 7 g Dietary Fiber 0 g Sugars 1 g Protein 23 g

JAMBALAYA

A hallmark of Creole cooking, jambalaya is a versatile dish that combines cooked rice with a variety of vegetables—such as tomatoes, onions, and green peppers—and almost any kind of meat, poultry, and shellfish. Jambalaya recipes vary from cook to cook and ingredients are often added depending upon what's at hand. Here's one of our favorite versions that's sure to become a favorite with you, too.

Number of Servings: 8   **Serving Size:** 1-1/4 cups

INGREDIENTS

Name	Measure/Weight
canola oil or corn oil	1 Tbsp
medium onion, chopped	2 ea
green bell pepper, cored and peeled	1 ea
celery, chopped	2 ea
clove garlic, minced	2 ea
can diced tomatoes in puree, undrained	16 oz
low-fat, low-sodium chicken broth	2 cups
tomato paste	2 Tbsp

salt	1 tsp
thyme	1 1/2 tsp
fresh ground black pepper	1/4 tsp
cayenne pepper	1/4 tsp
bay leaf	1 ea
hot pepper sauce	8 drops
uncooked long grain rice	1 1/2 cups
diced cooked ham	1 cup
boneless, skinless chicken breasts, cooked	1 cup
shrimp, peeled and deveined	6 oz

PREPARATION INSTRUCTIONS

1. Heat the oil in a large, heavy pot. Add the onions, green pepper, celery, and garlic and sauté over medium heat until softened.
2. Add the tomatoes and liquid, the chicken broth, tomato paste, and seasonings; simmer, uncovered, for 10 minutes.
3. Add the rice; cover and simmer for 10 minutes. Add the ham and chicken. Continue cooking, covered, for 10 to 15 minutes, or until the rice absorbs the liquid. Stir to mix well. Add the shrimp for the last 3 minutes of cooking. Remove the bay leaf before serving.

Exchanges Per Serving	*Nutrition Information Amount per serving*	
2 Starch	Calories 263	Sodium 658 mg
2 Vegetable	Calories From Fat 40	Total Carbohydrate 37 g
1 Meat Lean	Total Fat 4 g	Dietary Fiber 2 g
	Saturated Fat 1 g	Sugars 5 g
	Cholestrol 56 mg	Protein 18 g

LIME-GRILLED FISH WITH FRESH SALSA

Lime-grilled fish is a taste straight from sunny Mexico, and perfect for a backyard summer barbecue.

Number of Servings: 4 **Serving Size:** 1 fillet plus 1/4 cup salsa

INGREDIENTS

Name	Measure/Weight
olive oil	1 Tbsp
lime juice	1 Tbsp
firm fish fillets, such as orange roughy or red snapper (1 pound total) thawed, if frozen	4 ea
salsa	1 cup
lime cut into 4 slices	1/2 ea

PREPARATION INSTRUCTIONS

1. Prepare a charcoal grill, or preheat the broiler and prepare the broiler pan with nonstick cooking spray.
2. Combine the oil and lime juice; brush over the fish. Grill or broil 4 to 5 inches from the heat source until the fish is opaque, about 6 minutes (depending on the thickness of the fish). Serve immediately, topped with salsa and fresh lime slices.

Exchanges Per Serving	Nutrition Information Amount per serving	
1 Vegetable	Calories 164	Sodium 356 mg
3 Meat Very Lean	Calories From Fat 46	Total Carbohydrate 5 g
1/2 Monounsaturated	Total Fat 5 g	Dietary Fiber 1 g
Fat	Saturated Fat 1 g	Sugars 3 g
	Cholestrol 42 mg	Protein 24 g

SEASONED PAN-FRIED CATFISH

A delicious entrée for the whole family

Number of Servings: 4   **Serving Size:** 4 oz

INGREDIENTS

Name	Measure/Weight
potato flakes, instant	1/2 cup
salt, seasoned	1/2 tsp
pepper, ground black	1/8 tsp
catfish fillets	1 lb
egg, beaten	1 ea
cooking spray, butter-flavored	1 spray

PREPARATION INSTRUCTIONS

1. In a shallow dish, combine potato flakes, seasoned salt, and pepper. Dip catfish fillets in beaten egg, then coat well with seasoned potato mixture.
2. Place in a large nonstick skillet coated generously with non-stick cooking spray, and cook over medium heat until fillets are golden, about 10 minutes.
3. Spray remaining uncooked side of fillets with cooking spray, turn over, and continue cooking until golden and fish flakes easily with a fork (about 10 more minutes). Turn only once during cooking.

Exchanges Per Serving	Nutrition Information Amount per serving	
4 Very Lean Meat	Calories 165	Sodium 233 mg
1/2 Starch	Calories From Fat 45	Total Carbohydrate 7 g
	Total Fat 5 g	Dietary Fiber 1 g
	Saturated Fat 1 g	Sugars 0 g
	Cholestrol 158 mg	Protein 23 g

TUNA RICE PIE

Here's an easy and tasty solution for last-minute dinners—you probably have most of the ingredients in your cupboard.

Number of Servings: 6　　　　　**Serving Size:** 1 wedge

INGREDIENTS

Name	Measure/Weight
uncooked long grain rice	1/3 cup
salt	1/4 tsp
margarine	1 tsp
egg, or 1/2 cup egg substitute	2 ea
can water-packed tuna or salmon, drained and flaked	6 1/2 oz
milk, fat-free (skim)	3/4 cup
fresh or thawed frozen peas	1 1/2 cups
parsley	1 Tbsp
freshly ground pepper	1/4 tsp
nutmeg	1/8 tsp
slices reduced-fat Swiss or Colby	4 slices

LIVING WITH DIABETES

Preparation Instructions

1. Preheat the oven to 350 degrees F. Prepare a 9-inch pie pan with nonstick cooking spray.
2. Combine the rice, 1 cup water, and the salt in a small saucepan; bring to a boil, cover, and simmer 14 minutes. Separate the rice grains with a fork.
3. Beat 1 egg in a small bowl. Stir the margarine and beaten egg into the rice mixture. Press the rice against the sides and bottom of the pie pan to make crust. Spread the tuna or salmon evenly over the rice.
4. In a saucepan, heat the milk and peas to a simmer. Add the parsley, pepper, and nutmeg. Beat the remaining egg and stir into the milk mixture. Pour over the tuna.
5. Layer slices of cheese over the top. Bake for about 25 minutes. Cut the pie in 6 equal wedges.

Exchanges Per Serving	*Nutrition Information Amount per serving*	
1 Starch	Calories 190	Sodium 322 mg
2 Lean Meat	Calories From Fat 45	Total Carbohydrate 16 g
	Total Fat 5 g	Dietary Fiber 2 g
	Saturated Fat 2 g	Sugars 4 g
	Cholestrol 86 mg	Protein 19 g

CREAMY BLUE CHEESE DRESSING

Rich and creamy for salad greens or vegetable dips.

Number of Servings: 12   **Serving Size:** 2 Tbsp

INGREDIENTS

Name	*Measure/Weight*
low-fat cottage cheese	1 cup
blue cheese, crumbled	2 Tbsp
fat-free milk	3 Tbsp
garlic clove squeezed through garlic press	1 ea

PREPARATION INSTRUCTIONS

1. Place the cottage cheese, blue cheese, and milk in a blender or food processor.
2. Push the garlic through a garlic press into the work bowl. Process for about 20 seconds. (The blue cheese should still be chunky.)
3. Keeps for 1 week in a tightly covered jar in the refrigerator.

Exchanges Per Serving	*Nutrition Information Amount per serving*	
1/2 Lean Meat	Calories 25	Sodium 103 mg
	Calories From Fat 9	Total Carbohydrate 2 g
	Total Fat 1 g	Dietary Fiber 0 g
	Saturated Fat 1 g	Sugars 0 g
	Cholestrol 4 mg	Protein 3 g

BOLOGNESE SAUCE

This traditional Italian meat sauce is a snap to make and freezes well. Make a big batch so you always have some on hand. Use it as a base sauce for lasagna or ladle some over any shape of pasta, from angel hair to ziti.

Number of Servings: 4　　　　**Serving Size:** 3/4 cup

INGREDIENTS

Name	*Measure/Weight*
90 percent lean ground beef	3/4 lb
chopped onion	1/2 cup
clove garlic, minced	1 ea
carrot, coarsely chopped	1/4 cup
can diced tomatoes in puree, undrained	16 oz
dry red wine	1/4 cup
chopped fresh basil	1 Tbsp
chopped fresh oregano	2 tsp
salt	3/4 tsp
fresh ground black pepper	1/8 tsp
tomato paste	1 Tbsp

PREPARATION INSTRUCTIONS

1. Brown the ground beef in a large nonstick skillet with the onion, garlic, and carrot over medium heat; drain off the fat and return the beef and vegetables to the skillet.
2. Add the tomatoes with their liquid, the wine, and the seasonings and herbs. Cover and simmer for 40 to 45 minutes, stirring occasionally.
3. Stir in the tomato paste; simmer, uncovered for 5 to 10 minutes, until slightly thickened.

Exchanges Per Serving	Nutrition Information Amount per serving	
2 Vegetable	Calories 203	Sodium 694 mg
3 Lean Meat	Calories From Fat 79	Total Carbohydrate 9 g
	Total Fat 9 g	Dietary Fiber 2 g
	Saturated Fat 3 g	Sugars 5 g
	Cholestrol 63 mg	Protein 22 g

Copyright © American Diabetes Association
From *The New Family Cookbook for People With Diabetes*

CRISPY BAKED CHICKEN

Cornflake crumbs give this skinless chicken a crisp coating even in the microwave oven. Energy-saving tip: The most energy-efficient way to cook small amounts of meat is in the microwave.

Number of Servings: 2   **Serving Size:** 2 ounces

INGREDIENTS

Name	Measure/Weight
boneless, skinless chicken breast, split	1 ea
low-fat (1%) milk	1/4 cup
cornflakes crumbs	1/4 cup
chopped fresh rosemary or coriander	1/4 tsp
pepper	1 pinch

PREPARATION INSTRUCTIONS

1. Rinse and dry chicken pieces thoroughly. Dip in milk.
2. Mix cornflake crumbs with rosemary or coriander and pepper. Roll chicken in the seasoned crumbs.

3. Place on microwave-safe roasting rack. Cover with paper towel.
4. Microwave 4-6 minutes on High or until done.

Exchanges Per Serving	Nutrition Information Amount per serving	
2 Lean Meat	Calories 106	Sodium 119 mg
	Calories From Fat 18	Total Carbohydrate 4 g
	Total Fat 2 g	Dietary Fiber 0 g
	Saturated Fat 0 g	Sugars 0 g
	Cholestrol 60 mg	Protein 18 g

Copyright © American Diabetes Association
From *The Healthy HomeStyle Cookbook*

BAKED ACORN SQUASH WITH APPLE STUFFING

Acorn squash is the most common member of the winter squash family. Its bright orange flesh bakes beautifully, coming out moist, rich, and tender, and its pretty dark green and orange-streaked shell makes a perfect container for the delicious apple stuffing.

Number of Servings: 4   **Serving Size:** 1/2 squash

INGREDIENTS

Name	Measure/Weight
small acorn squash, halved and seeded	2 ea
apples, peeled and diced	1 ea
celery, diced	2 Tbsp
onion, finely chopped	2 Tbsp
margarine, melted	2 tsp

APPENDIX: DELICIOUS AND HEALTHY RECIPES

salt   1 pinch
fresh ground black pepper   1 pinch

PREPARATION INSTRUCTIONS

1. Preheat the oven to 400 degrees F. Prepare a square baking pan with nonstick cooking spray.
2. Place the squash cut side down in a baking pan. Bake for 20 minutes.
3. While the squash is baking, combine the apples, celery, onion, margarine, and 2 tablespoons water in a medium bowl; mix well.
4. Turn the squash cut sides up. Sprinkle with salt and pepper. Divide the apple mixture to fill the cavities of the squash. Bake the stuffed squash halves, covered with foil, for 30 minutes more. Serve hot.

Exchanges Per Serving	*Nutrition Information Amount per serving*	
1 Starch	Calories 87	Sodium 63 mg
	Calories From Fat 19	Total Carbohydrate 18 g
	Total Fat 2 g	Dietary Fiber 5 g
	Saturated Fat 0 g	Sugars 10 g
	Cholestrol 0 mg	Protein 1 g

Copyright © American Diabetes Association
From *The New Family Cookbook for People With Diabetes*

VEGETABLE LASAGNA

A hearty, delicious meal that's perfect for entertaining

Number of Servings: 6   **Serving Size:** 1 cup

INGREDIENTS

Name	*Measure/Weight*
sliced carrot	1 cup
sliced zucchini	1 cup
diced red pepper	1/2 cup
chopped spinach	1 cup
low-fat cottage cheese	1 cup
part-skim ricotta cheese	1/2 cup
egg substitute	2 ea
minced fresh basil	1 tsp
minced fresh oregano	1 tsp
fresh ground pepper to taste	1 pinch
low-fat, low-sodium marinara sauce	2 cups
uncooked lasagna noodles	9 ea

PREPARATION INSTRUCTIONS

1. To prepare the vegetables, steam the carrots over boiling water for 2 minutes. Add the zucchini and steam 2 more minutes. Add the red pepper and steam 2 more minutes. Add the spinach and steam 1 more minute. Remove the vegetables from the heat. Combine all remaining ingredients except the marinara sauce and lasagna noodles.

2. To assemble the lasagna, place a little sauce on the bottom of a casserole dish. Place 3 noodles on top of the sauce. Add a layer of vegetables and cover with a layer of the cheese mix-

ture. Add some sauce. Repeat. Add the last layer of noodles and top with some sauce. Refrigerate overnight. The next day, preheat the oven to 350 degrees F. Bake the lasagna for 40 minutes until bubbly. Let stand 10 minutes prior to serving. Cut into squares and serve. (If you prefer to bake the lasagna immediately, cook the pasta before layering it.)

Exchanges Per Serving	Nutrition Information Amount per serving	
3 Starch	Calories 271	Total Carbohydrates
1 Very Lean Meat	Calories From Fat 16	46 g
	Total Fat 2 g	Dietary Fiber 4 g
	Saturated Fat 1 g	Sugars 11 g
	Cholestrol 10 mg	Protein 18 g
	Sodium 520 mg	

Copyright © American Diabetes Association
From *Flavorful Seasons Cookbook* by Robyn Webb

SMOTHERED BAKED PORTABELLO MUSHROOM

An unusual and mouth-watering dish!

Number of Servings: 1   **Serving Size:** 1

INGREDIENTS

Name	Measure/Weight
large cap portabello mushroom	1 ea
low-fat ricotta cheese	2 Tbsp
garlic powder	1/4 tsp
black pepper	1/4 tsp
cooked pasta (linguini, spaghetti, or fettcuine)	1 cup

| tomato sauce | 1/2 cup |
| shredded mozzarella cheese, part skim | 1/4 cup |

Preparation Instructions

1. Heat oven to 350 degrees F. Stem mushroom and sauté in nonstick pan 2-3 minutes on each side.
2. Spoon ricotta cheese into mushroom cavity and sprinkle with garlic powder and pepper.
3. Place pasta in a shallow nonstick baking dish. Pour 1/2 cup sauce over pasta. Place mushroom cap side up on top of pasta.
4. Pour remaining sauce over mushroom and sprinkle with cheese. Bake 20 minutes or until cheese bubbles.

Exchanges Per Serving	*Nutrition Information Amount per serving*	
4 Starch	Calories 413	Sodium 232 mg
1 Lean Meat	Calories From Fat 71	Total Carbohydrate 71 g
2 Vegetable	Total Fat 8 g	Dietary Fiber 8 g
	Saturated Fat 4 g	Sugars 17 g
	Cholestrol 28 mg	Protein 23 g

OATMEAL RAISIN COOKIES

These oatmeal raisin cookies are packed with flavor and have only 2 grams of fat per cookie. They'll keep in an airtight container up to 1 week or in the freezer for up to 1 month.

Number of Servings: 20   **Serving Size:** 2 cookies

APPENDIX: DELICIOUS AND HEALTHY RECIPES

Ingredients

Name	Measure/Weight
all-purpose flour	1 cup
baking powder	1/2 tsp
baking soda	1/2 tsp
cinnamon	3/4 tsp
salt	1/4 tsp
stick margarine	5 Tbsp
granulated sugar	1/4 cup
firmly packed light brown sugar	1/4 cup
egg	1 ea
low-fat (1%) milk	1/4 cup
pure vanilla extract	1 tsp
quick-cooking oats	2 1/4 cups
seedless raisins	1/3 cup

Preparation Instructions

1. Preheat the oven to 375 degrees F. Line a baking sheet with parchment paper or spray with nonstick cooking spray.
2. In a small bowl, whisk together the flour, baking powder, baking soda, cinnamon, and salt. Set aside.
3. In a medium bowl, with an electric mixer on medium speed, beat the margarine until creamy, 2 minutes. Gradually blend in the sugars. Add the egg and continue beating until smooth, 1 minute. Beat in the milk and vanilla until smooth. Add the flour mixture to the margarine mixture in thirds, and blend until smooth, 2 minutes. Stir in the oats and raisins.
4. Drop the dough by teaspoonfuls onto the prepared baking sheet. Bake until lightly browned, about 7-9 minutes. With a spatula, remove the cookies to a rack and cool completely.

Exchanges Per Serving	Nutrition Information Amount per serving	
1 Carbohydrate	Calories 115	Sodium 109 mg
1 Fat	Calories From Fat 34	Total Carbohydrate 18 g
	Total Fat 4 g	Dietary Fiber 1 g
	Saturated Fat 1 g	Sugars 7 g
	Cholestrol 11 mg	Protein 3 g

APPLESAUCE MUFFINS

Applesauce makes the muffins tender and moist without overloading them with fat.

Number of Servings: 12   **Serving Size:** 1 muffin

INGREDIENTS

Name	Measure/Weight
unsweetened applesauce	1 1/4 cups
egg	1 ea
canola or corn oil	2 Tbsp
honey	1/4 cup
whole-wheat flour	1 cup
all-purpose flour	1 cup
baking powder	2 tsp
baking soda	3/4 tsp
cinnamon	1/2 tsp
nutmeg	1/4 tsp
raisins	1/3 cup

PREPARATION INSTRUCTIONS

1. Preheat oven to 375 degrees F. In a large bowl, beat together the applesauce, egg, oil, and honey.
2. Sift in the dry ingredients; stirring just to moisten.
3. Stir in the raisins and divide the batter among 12 muffin cups coated with nonstick cooking spray.
4. Bake for 20 minutes.

Exchanges Per Serving	Nutrition Information Amount per serving	
1 Starch	Calories 143	Sodium 130 mg
1 Fruit	Calories From Fat 27	Total Carbohydrate 26 g
1/2 Fat	Total Fat 3 g	Dietary Fiber 2 g
	Saturated Fat 0 g	Sugars 0 g
	Cholestrol 18 mg	Protein 3 g

DELUXE CARROT CAKE

Serve thin slices for a large gathering that has eaten a hearty main course. Serve thick slabs to fewer people who have had a rather light entreé. Pass Maple/Yogurt Sauce if desired: Stir together 1/2 cup low-fat plain yogurt, 2 tsp maple syrup, and a couple drops of vanilla and chill.

Number of Servings: 16   **Serving Size:** 1 slice

INGREDIENTS

Name	Measure/Weight
crushed pinapple in unsweetened juice, divided and drained	20 oz

all-purpose flour	2 cups
non-fat powdered milk	1 cup
baking powder	2 tsp
cinnamon	2 tsp
walnuts, roughly chopped	1/2 cup
shredded carrots	2 cups
egg substitute	3/4 cup
canola or corn oil	1/3 cup
vanilla	2 tsp
unsweetened coconut	1 cup
raisins	3/4 cup
low-fat ricotta cheese	1 cup
artificial sweetener	4 pkg
vanilla	2 tsp

PREPARATION INSTRUCTIONS

1. Preheat oven to 350 degrees F. Drain juice from pineapple. Reserve one half of the drained pineapples for the filling and frosting.
2. Sift together the flour, powdered milk, baking powder, and cinnamon.
3. Add the walnuts and carrots.
4. In a separate bowl, mix together eggs, juice, oil and vanilla.
5. Blend the two mixtures together until just combined. Fold in 1 cup drained pineapple, coconut, and raisins.
6. Pour into two 9-inch round cake pans that have been coated with nonstick cooking spray and floured. Bake for 40 minutes. Let cool 10 minutes in pans, then remove and cool completely on racks before frosting.

7. For the Frosting; beat ricotta, sweetener, and vanilla until fluffy, then stir in pineapple. Spread between layers.

Exchanges Per Serving	Nutrition Information Amount per serving	
2 Starch	Calories 262	Sodium 142 mg
2 Fat	Calories From Fat 90	Total Carbohydrate 32 g
	Total Fat 10 g	Dietary Fiber 1 g
	Saturated Fat 3 g	Sugars 0 g
	Cholestrol 2 mg	Protein 11 g

BLUE CHEESE VEGETABLE ROLL-UP

A great snack for company!

Number of Servings: 1   **Serving Size: 1 tortilla**

INGREDIENTS

Name	Measure/Weight
whole-wheat or corn tortillas	1 ea
low-fat blue cheese dressing	1 Tbsp
4-inch celery sticks	2 ea
4-inch carrot sticks	2 ea

PREPARATION INSTRUCTIONS

1. Heat tortilla per package directions.
2. Spread dressing on tortilla, add celery and carrot sticks to end of tortilla, and roll up.

Exchanges Per Serving	*Nutrition Information Amount per serving*	
2 Starch	Calories 234	Sodium 442 mg
1 Vegetable	Calories From Fat 65	Total Carbohydrate 36 g
1 Fat	Total Fat 7 g	Dietary Fiber 3 g
	Saturated Fat 2 g	Sugars 3 g
	Cholestrol 1 mg	Protein 6 g

CARAMEL CRUNCH POPCORN

In this recipe, a little caramel flavor goes a long way. Although the serving size is small, there's plenty of satisfying sweet taste and crunchy texture. This recipe makes a big batch and can be stored in an airtight container and kept for about 1 week.

Number of Servings: 24   **Serving Size:** 1/2 cup

INGREDIENTS

Name	*Measure/Weight*
plain air-popped popcorn (about 1 cup unpopped)	12 cups
granulated sugar	1 cup
stick margarine	10 Tbsp
light corn syrup	1/3 cup
vanilla extract	1 tsp

PREPARATION INSTRUCTIONS

1. Cover 2 baking sheets with aluminum foil and spray with nonstick cooking spray. Spread the popped popcorn on the baking sheets in a single layer.

2. In a medium nonstick skillet, combine the sugar, margarine, and syrup. Bring to a boil over medium heat, stirring constantly, about 3 minutes. Continue cooking and stirring until the mixture turns a light caramel color, 5 minutes; do not overcook or the caramel will brown and burn! Remove from the heat and slowly stir in the vanilla.

3. Pour the caramel mixture over the popcorn. When the caramel has cooled, break it into bite-sized pieces.

Exchanges Per Serving	Nutrition Information Amount per serving	
1 Carbohydrate	Calories 109	Sodium 63 mg
1 Fat	Calories From Fat 44	Total Carbohydrate 17 g
	Total Fat 5 g	Dietary Fiber 1 g
	Saturated Fat 1 g	Sugars 12 g
	Cholestrol 0 mg	Protein 0 g

Copyright © American Diabetes Association
From *Forbidden Foods Diabetic Cooking*

NACHOS

The secret to lighter nachos? Look for low-fat tortilla chips with only 2 grams of fat per serving, then focus on adding flavorful vegetables rather than extra cheese. Green chiles, tomatoes, green onions, and jalapeño peppers give them their pizzazz.

Number of Servings: 6   **Serving Size:** 3/4 cup

INGREDIENTS

Name	Measure/Weight
low-fat baked tortilla chips	4 cups
grated extra sharp cheddar cheese	1 cup

canned chopped green chilies	2 Tbsp
medium tomato, finely chopped	1/2 ea
sliced black olives	1/4 cup
green onion, finely chopped	1 ea
chopped cilantro	2 Tbsp
pickled jalapeño peppers, sliced (optional)	2 ea

PREPARATION INSTRUCTIONS

1. Preheat the oven to 400 degrees F. Spray a large heatproof platter or baking sheet with nonstick cooking spray.
2. Scatter the tortilla chips evenly over the platter. Sprinkle then evenly with the cheese and green chiles and broil until the cheese melts, 2-3 minutes.
3. Top the nachos with the chopped tomato, olives, cilantro, and the jalapeño peppers, if using. Serve immediately.

Exchanges Per Serving	*Nutrition Information Amount per serving*	
1 Starch	Calories 172	Sodium 319 mg
1 Lean Meat	Calories From Fat 79	Total Carbohydrate 18 g
1 Fat	Total Fat 9 g	Dietary Fiber 3 g
	Saturated Fat 4 g	Sugars 1 g
	Cholestrol 20 mg	Protein 7 g

OVEN-FRIED ONION RINGS

Light and tasty treats are particularly sweet with Vidalia onions but are good with whatever is available.

Number of Servings: 4   **Serving Size:** 1/2 cup (2 oz)

INGREDIENTS

Name	Measure/Weight
Vidalia onion, thinly sliced	1 ea
reduced-calorie corn oil	1 Tbsp
cornmeal	2 Tbsp
fine bread crumbs	2 Tbsp
Parmesan cheese	1 Tbsp
paprika	1/8 tsp

PREPARATION INSTRUCTIONS

1. Peel onion; slice into 1/4 inch rings.
2. Sprinkle with oil and toss to coat.
3. Mix dry ingredients, sprinkle over onion rings, and toss to coat evenly.
4. Place on a nonstick baking sheet. Bake at 400 degrees for 20 minutes or until lightly browned.

Exchanges Per Serving	Nutrition Information Amount per serving	
2 Vegetable	Calories 93	Sodium 104 mg
1 Fat	Calories From Fat 45	Total Carbohydrate 9 g
	Total Fat 5 g	Dietary Fiber 1 g
	Saturated Fat 1 g	Sugars 0 g
	Cholestrol 3 mg	Protein 3 g

TOAST AND JAM TREAT

Number of Servings: 1   **Serving Size:** 1 piece

INGREDIENTS

Name	Measure/Weight
low-fat cottage cheese	1/4 cup
jam, low sugar	2 Tbsp
non-fat powdered milk	1 Tbsp
bread, toasted	1 slice

PREPARATION INSTRUCTIONS

1. In a blender or food processor, combine cottage cheese, jam, and dry, powdered milk and spread on toast.

Exchanges Per Serving	Nutrition Information Amount per serving	
1 Starch	Calories 168	Sodium 389 mg
1 Very Lean Meat	Calories From Fat 14	Total Carbohydrate 28 g
1 Fruit	Total Fat 2 g	Dietary Fiber 1 g
	Saturated Fat 0 g	Sugars 10 g
	Cholestrol 3 mg	Protein 10 g

ZUCCHINI PIZZAS

For the adventurous vegetable lovers out there.

Number of Servings: 10   **Serving Size:** 3 slices

INGREDIENTS

Name	Measure/Weight
zucchini, about 2 inches in diameter, cut into 1/4-inch slices	2 ea
pizza sauce	1 Tbsp
pitted black olives, sliced	1 tsp
green onion minced	1 tsp
fat-free mozzarella, grated	2 Tbsp

PREPARATION INSTRUCTIONS

1. On each slice of zucchini place ingredients in order.
2. Place on a baking sheet and broil until cheese is melted and bubbly, about 3-5 minutes. Zucchini should be crisp.

Exchanges Per Serving	Nutrition Information Amount per serving	
1 Lean Meat	Calories 53	Sodium 373 mg
	Calories From Fat 9	Total Carbohydrate 5 g
	Total Fat 1 g	Dietary Fiber 1 g
	Saturated Fat 0 g	Sugars 0 g
	Cholestrol 1 mg	Protein g

HONEY LAMB CHOPS

Mustard and honey flavor these lamb chops.

Number of Servings: 6   **Serving Size:** 3 oz

INGREDIENTS

Name	*Measure/Weight*
honey	2 Tbsp
fresh lemon juice	2 Tbsp
minced fresh rosemary	2 Tbsp
Dijon mustard	1/2 tsp
minced garlic	1 tsp
onion powder	1 tsp
dry mustard	1/2 tsp
5-oz lamb chops, trimmed of fat	6 slices
sprigs fresh mint	6 sprigs

PREPARATION INSTRUCTIONS

1. Combine all ingredients except the lamb chops and mint in a small bowl and microwave for 1 minute.
2. Brush the mixture on the chops and broil or grill, turning frequently, according to the following guidelines: 12 minutes for rare, 15 minutes for medium, and 18 minutes for well done.
3. Garnish with mint and serve.

Exchanges Per Serving	Nutrition Information Amount per serving	
2 Meat Lean	Calories 139	Sodium 45 mg
1/2 Starch	Calories From Fat 54	Total Carbohydrate 5 g
	Total Fat 6 g	Dietary Fiber 0 g
	Saturated Fat 2 g	Sugars 5 g
	Cholestrol 52 mg	Protein 16 g

Copyright © American Diabetes Association

From *Flavorful Seasons Cookbook* by **Robyn Webb**

POWER BURGER

A delicious, healthy meal!

Number of Servings: 2   **Serving Size:** 1 burger

INGREDIENTS

Name	Measure/Weight
90 percent lean ground beef	1/2 lb
oat bran	2 Tbsp
oats	1/4 cup
fat-free milk	2 Tbsp
dehydrated minced onion	1 tsp
pepper	1 dash
canola or corn oil	1/2 tsp

PREPARATION INSTRUCTIONS

1. Mix all ingredients together except oil and form into 2 patties. Heat oil in skillet and cook burgers until done.

Exchanges Per Serving	Nutrition Information Amount per serving	
1 Starch	Calories 296	Sodium 73 mg
3 Medium Fat Meat	Calories From Fat 153	Total Carbohydrate 11 g
	Total Fat 17 g	Dietary Fiber 2 g
	Saturated Fat 6 g	Sugars 1 g
	Cholestrol 71 mg	Protein 23 g

WINTER BEEF STEW

Pears and apples, winter's finest fruits, compliment lean beef in this hearty stew.

Number of Servings: 6 **Serving Size:** 1 cup with 3-4 oz beef

INGREDIENTS

Name	Measure/Weight
canola oil	1 Tbsp
chopped onion	1 cup
garlic cloves, minced	3 ea
carrots, cut into 1-inch slices	2 ea
lean stew beef, cut into 1-inch cubes	1 1/2 lb
low-fat, low-sodium beef broth	3 cups
paprika	1 tsp
Fresh ground pepper and salt to taste	1 pinch
mixed pears and apples, unpeeled and chopped into 1-inch pieces	1 1/2 cups

APPENDIX: DELICIOUS AND HEALTHY RECIPES

PREPARATION INSTRUCTIONS

1. Heat the oil in a large stockpot over medium-high heat. Add the onion and garlic and sauté for 5 minutes. Add the carrots and sauté for another 5 minutes. Add the meat and brown. Drain off any accumulated fat. Add the broth, paprika, pepper and salt (if desired).
2. Bring to a boil over high heat. Reduce the heat and simmer, uncovered, for 1-1/4 hours. Add the apples and pears and cover. Cook over low heat for 15-20 minutes until the apples and pears are soft, but not mushy.

Exchanges Per Serving	*Nutrition Information Amount per serving*	
1 Starch	Calories 223	Sodium 156 mg
3 Very Lean Meat	Calories From Fat 69	Total Carbohydrate 14 g
1 Monounsaturated	Total Fat 8 g	Dietary Fiber 3 g
Fat	Saturated Fat 2 g	Sugars 9 g
	Cholestrol 59 mg	Protein 27 g

Copyright © American Diabetes Association
From *Flavorful Seasons Cookbook* by Robyn Webb

BREAKFAST QUESADILLAS

A different kind of breakfast treat!

Number of Servings: 2   **Serving Size:** 1/2 quesadilla

INGREDIENTS

Name	*Measure/Weight*
8-inch flour tortillas	2 ea

egg substitute	1/2 cup
black pepper	1 dash
cayenne pepper	1 dash
fresh tomato	2 slices
fat-free cheese	1 slice
onion, optional	1 slice

PREPARATION INSTRUCTIONS

1. Heat oven to 375 degrees F. Scramble egg substitute in small skillet.
2. Lay 1 tortilla on a nonstick baking sheet. Spoon cooked egg substitute on top and sprinkle with peppers. Top with tomato, cheese, and onion, if desired.
3. Add second tortilla on top. Press lightly. Bake 5 minutes, flip, and bake 5 more minutes or until cheese is melted. Cut into fourths to serve.

Exchanges Per Serving	*Nutrition Information Amount per serving*	
2 Starch	Calories 216	Sodium 451 mg
1 Lean Meat	Calories From Fat 33	Total Carbohydrate 30 g
	Total Fat 4 g	Dietary Fiber 2 g
	Saturated Fat 1 g	Sugars 3 g
	Cholestrol 2 mg	Protein 15 g

HONEY-MUSTARD CHICKEN WINGS

Chicken wings deliver a lot of flavor for a relatively low price.
A chicken drumette is the meaty drumstick section of the wing,
and drumettes can ordinarily be purchased frozen. If they are not
available, buy 2 pounds of whole chicken wings and cut each into
3 segments. Use the meaty section for this recipe and reserve the
tips for stock.

Number of Servings: 8   **Serving Size:** 2 drumettes

INGREDIENTS

Name	*Measure/Weight*
spicy brown mustard	2 Tbsp
honey	1 Tbsp plus 1 tsp
dry bread crumbs	1/3 cup
chicken wing drumettes (about 16 pieces)	1 1/2 lb
Hungarian paprika, preferably hot	1/4 tsp

PREPARATION INSTRUCTIONS

1. Preheat the oven to 375 degrees F. Spray cookie sheet with nonstick cooking spray.
2. Combine the mustard and honey in a small bowl. Place the bread crumbs in a separate shallow bowl. Brush each wing section with the mustard mixture. Roll each in bread crumbs; shake off excess.
3. Place the wings on the cookie sheet and sprinkle with paprika, if desired. Bake the wings 30 minutes, or until crispy. Serve warm.

Exchanges Per Serving	*Nutrition Information Amount per serving*	
1/2 Starch	Calories 129	Sodium 113 mg
1 Medium-Fat Meat	Calories From Fat 63	Total Carbohydrate 6 g
	Total Fat 7 g	Dietary Fiber 0 g
	Saturated Fat 2 g	Sugars 3 g
	Cholestrol 29 mg	Protein 10 g

BANANA SHAKES

This creamy shake takes just minutes to make and is ideal for a quick on-the-go breakfast or afternoon pick-me-up-with just 1 gram of fat. Experiment with other fruits for a change of flavor, substituting 1 cup of another fresh or frozen (no sugar added) fruit in place of the banana. Try pitted sweet Bing cherries, raspberries, strawberries, peaches, mango, or a combination of fruits.

Number of Servings: 2   **Serving Size:** 1 cup

INGREDIENTS

Name	*Measure/Weight*
fat-free milk	1 cup
vanilla low-fat frozen yogurt	1/2 cup
ripe banana, peeled	1 ea
pure vanilla extract	1/4 tsp

PREPARATION INSTRUCTIONS

1. Blend the milk and frozen yogurt in a blender or food processor about 1 minute.

2. Add the banana and vanilla; blend a few seconds longer.

Exchanges Per Serving	Nutrition Information Amount per serving	
1 Fruit	Calories 130	Sodium 83 mg
1/2 Milk, low-fat	Calories From Fat 10	Total Carbohydrate 24 g
	Total Fat 1 g	Dietary Fiber 1 g
	Saturated Fat 1 g	Sugars 17 g
	Cholestrol 7 mg	Protein 6 g

Copyright © American Diabetes Association. From *The New Family Cookbook for People With Diabetes.*

HOT CHOCOLATE

Brrrrr! Some days just call for hot chocolate. Although this recipe makes one serving, you can easily double or triple it when friends come by. Use the best quality unsweetened cocoa powder that you can find. For extra flavor, crush a small peppermint hard candy in the hot cocoa and stir to blend.

Number of Servings: 1   **Serving Size:** 1 cup

INGREDIENTS

Name	Measure/Weight
fat-free milk, heated	1 cup
powdered sugar	2 Tbsp
unsweetened cocoa powder	2 tsp
pure vanilla extract	1/8 tsp

Preparation Instructions

1. In a small saucepan, heat the milk over medium heat, stirring occasionally, until bubbles at the sides of the pan, 2 minutes. Whisk in the sugar, cocoa, and vanilla until smooth.

Exchanges Per Serving	Nutrition Information Amount per serving	
1 Carbohydrate	Calories 154	Sodium 126 mg
1 Fat-Free Milk	Calories From Fat 8	Total Carbohydrate 29 g
	Total Fat 1 g	Dietary Fiber 1 g
	Saturated Fat 0 g	Sugars 26 g
	Cholestrol 4 mg	Protein 9 g

INDEX

low blood sugar. *See* hypoglycemia

meal planning, 64–66. *See also*
diet and nutrition
stocking kitchen, 65–66
medical alert ID bracelet,
89–90, 100, 116
medications, 127–136. *See
also* insulin
fine-tuning your regimen,
130–131
questions to ask regarding,
131
knowing names of,
129–130
oral hypoglycemics,
132–136
side effects, 130
treatment advances, 172
when effective, 128–129
meglitinides (oral medication), 136
metabolic syndrome, 15,
109
metformin (oral medication),
134
side effects, 134
microalbumin test, 123,
152–153

Native Americans and dia-
betes, 14, 16
Pima Indians, 17–18
neuropathy, 153–155
symptoms of, 154–155
treatment for, 155
nurse educator, 114
nutrition. *See* diet and nutrition

obesity and diabetes, 15, 17
office visit to doctor, 122–125
ophthalmologist, 115, 150
oral hypoglycemics (medication), 132–136

pancreas, 1–3
function of, 1
transplantation, 171
Type 1 diabetes, 4
Type 2 diabetes, 5
patient's role in treatment,
116–126
meet with health care
providers, 119–120
stay on top of things,
121–125
talk to doctor, 117–119
peripheral neuropathy,
154–155

ABOUT THE AUTHORS

JAMES W. REED, M.D., M.A.C.P., F.A.C.E., was a member of the now defunct National Diabetes Advisory Board and is currently a member of the Education Council for the National Diabetes Educational Initiatives and the Diabetes Epidemic Action Council of the American Diabetes Association. He is Professor of Medicine and Associate Chair of Medicine for Research, Morehouse School of Medicine and a co-founder of the International Society for Hypertension in Blacks.

AGIUA HEATH, M.D., has been senior physician in Internal Medicine for Kaiser Permanente. At present, she is a physician with U.C. Berkeley Student Health Services.